30 YEARS
30,000 MILES

WHAT I LEARNED FROM GOD WHILE RUNNING

COLLEEN TRETTER

WESTBOW
PRESS®
A DIVISION OF THOMAS NELSON
& ZONDERVAN

Scripture taken from the Holy Bible, NEW INTERNATIONAL VERSION®. Copyright © 1973, 1978, 1984 by Biblica, Inc. All rights reserved worldwide. Used by permission. NEW INTERNATIONAL VERSION® and NIV® are registered trademarks of Biblica, Inc. Use of either trademark for the offering of goods or services requires the prior written consent of Biblica US, Inc.

WestBow Press books may be ordered through booksellers or by contacting:

WestBow Press
A Division of Thomas Nelson & Zondervan
1663 Liberty Drive
Bloomington, IN 47403
www.westbowpress.com
1 (866) 928-1240

ISBN: 978-1-4908-9900-8 (sc)
ISBN: 978-1-4908-9901-5 (hc)
ISBN: 978-1-4908-9899-5 (e)

Library of Congress Control Number: 2015911302

Print information available on the last page.

WestBow Press rev. date: 09/04/2015

For my five favorite runners,
Jim, my love, (and still my partner- even though
you don't run with me anymore),
Paul, my greatest protector,
Case, my greatest entertainer,
Cooper, my greatest encourager,
Timothy, my greatest healer.
I love you guys.
ECOHIH
cmast

PREFACE

This manuscript was not written to sell books. It was meant to result in one book only. So if your name isn't "Paul Tretter," my oldest son who called "dibs" on the "book" then God had other plans. You see, it took years of stalling, false starts, and stopping mid-stride in writing my journey, because I tried to convince God to raise up someone else who was better equipped to do it.

As one who is not any of the following: 1) an established author, 2) a professional runner and 3) a theologian, my prayer was that the person who met all three criteria would emerge to the starting line. In the meantime, God continued to lay the project on my heart. So I would acquiesce and write a few chapters, all the while waiting for the perfect tri-fecta candidate to show up.

I started running long distances in 1981 as a 16 year-old. As the years went by, so did life's milestones, including high school, college, joining Penn State's Army ROTC program, marriage, a career as a Registered Nurse, buying a farm and motherhood. Throughout those years, running persisted as the one constant through my journey in life. As I began to study scripture related to all God reveals about running, including paths and stumbling, my heart would beat with a pounding, not unlike what I experience in a quilt shop, or a cooking store. It was similar to the feeling when I felt I had perfected a crème brulee* recipe that was no fail, simple, and not too "egg-y tasting." Still, I yearned for someone best equipped to tell the story even as I felt gently prodded to tell mine.

After all, I don't even keep a continuous tally of my mileage, even though I do jot down each run.

A few more years passed of countless blessings of what God was revealing and yet still this project was a series of stops and starts. I felt like

Cameron in the movie, *Ferris Bueller's Day Off,* when he is sitting in the car at the beginning of the movie saying that Ferris will just keep bugging him until he goes saying, "I'll go. I'll go. I'll go. I'll go. I'll go. I'll go." Then he jumps out of the car and plans to *not go*! Not to equate God with Ferris Bueller, but I knew He (God) would keep bugging me until I finished it. So as my 50th birthday approached, I would sooner die than not get it done. Now that I have, I am grateful that God, in his great mercy, did not give me what I deserved which was a lightning bolt to my tush.

What He did allow was a herniated disc, which escalated slowly at first, and then rapidly just before Thanksgiving. All the while, I spent nights awake in pain deciding that I may as well do *something* which usually involved stringing Christmas lights then collapsing on the ottoman in various positions (on the floor legs up), face down, heat pack and stimulator on full blast, etc. The kids would awaken to the scene from Elf when Buddy prepared the department store for Santa's arrival.

When my entire right leg went numb, my husband alerted the neurosurgeon (I think he was alarmed that I would soon be in diapers), resulting in somewhat urgent surgery. With a lifting restriction of "nothing heavier than a Sunday paper," for me to finish the manuscript and thanks to my dear friend, Muff Dunlap, weeks of meals were brought to feed the troops, including my husband, four teenage boys and ten year-old. Add assistance with laundry (for four wrestlers no less) and care of my horses and dogs; I was compelled to sit under the Christmas tree and finish the manuscript.

As noted in Chapter 4, there was a time I lived to run, but I no longer live to run, which is probably another reason why I thought someone who did would be the best candidate to write this book. I run to *live*. My life is more defined by what I can do because of the running than running itself.

For some running is nothing more than a means to an end. And that is enough. But perhaps this book might change their perspective. At a recent luncheon, my dibs-calling son, Paul and I recently sat next to one of his most influential mentors, Pennsylvania State Police Trooper Jeffrey Brock, Director of Camp Cadet of Somerset County, an outstanding camp for teenagers. Trooper Brock was unaware that I had written a book about running, and as he was discussing the necessity of running at Camp Cadet and the State Police Academy, he told my son, "I *hate* to run. I absolutely hate it. But I do it." I chuckled to myself and thought, *and your life and the lives of countless others, including my own sons, are better because you do it.*

For others running is embraced because of how it enhances a more beloved sport, such as it does for our local wrestlers and soccer players. These athletes used their stamina to volunteer in a community project in 2012 to build a soccer field in our Community Park. Under the leadership of one of our extraordinary wrestling coaches-by-winter and groundskeeper-by-summer, Patsy Codispoti, the labor of love involved months of work. The sod that was donated by Oakbrook, one of our local golf courses, had to be cut into one-foot by three-foot pieces. Then the pieces were rolled, loaded onto a flatbed (they're heavier than you think!), unloaded, and pieced together on the prepped land. When I drive by that beautiful lush soccer field on Route 30, it warms my heart to see the legacy created by a bunch of filthy athletes.

And then there are those who cannot run at all, and yet they still understand the race of life better than others. When I returned from my summer at Walter Reed Army Medical Center in 1985 as an Army cadet nurse, I needed to find an apartment for my fall semester at Hershey Medical Center. An ad at the hospital stated, "Female Quadriplegic seeks nursing student. Free room in exchange for feeding supper, putting to bed, weekend assistance." I called and my life was never the same after meeting Nancy Euston. Most of my experience with people in wheelchairs up to that point involved elderly patients, and I'm a loud communicator to begin with, so one of the first things she told me was "I'm paralyzed, not deaf." Her paralysis was from the neck down, but she lived to her fullest, drawing sketches utilizing a pen in her mouth, which I still treasure. I still remember the time I admired her acceptance most when I returned from a run and turned on the shower, while she waited for me to bathe her. I cried and cried under that water. She couldn't run but she was running the race.

It's the beautiful extraordinary people about whom I feel compelled to testify that gave me real courage to complete this manuscript. My ordinary path had intertwined with those remarkable folks and extraordinary events in a unique way that can only be told by me. It would have been a crying shame to go to my *finish line* without having done so. When I finished this book planning a different title, this title came to me in the middle of the night. My first thought when I awoke was, "Have I actually run for thirty years and thirty thousand miles?" When I tallied the totals through the years, indeed I had.

My prayer is that everyone, runner and non-runner alike, would see what God is trying to reveal to them through people they encounter and in whatever activities they are engaged, whether art or photography or sports. My thirty-year journey (I exclude three years, allotting for my full term pregnancies, surgeries and illnesses) is fraught with full-blown stumbles, heart-wrenching mourning, joyous celebration, and simple contentment. Such is the nature of living. Sometimes it's the simplest events that no one knows about but God that connects us on the deepest levels.

On my wedding day, I took a short symbolic jaunt in the snow around my old high school. After a short while, I noticed a familiar set of shoe prints and step for step, my feet landed in them. At the reception, I asked my husband if he ran at the high school that morning and sure enough he had. He asked, "How did you know?" We had the same stride.

From the green hills of Ireland (we ran on the day of the Tiananmen Square massacre), to the black sandy beaches of Maui, the mileposts of life were marked by memories along the road. From the Golden Gate Bridge of San Francisco to the Brooklyn Bridge leading to our home in Long Island, life never stopped teaching something new.

From runs in Toronto to Orlando to San Antonio to Toledo, if all I learned in life were to try to be healthy, it would have been sufficient. But as I sought after and pursued God, my discovery was that all along He was pursuing me. From Colorado to Cleveland, from Johnstown to Jamaica, Washington D.C. to Washington State, as I ran, discovering that I was never alone and never forsaken, the real journey began for me. I hope it does for you as well. C.T.

*Colleen's Super Simple Crème Brulee Recipe

(Need ramekins and a kitchen torch)
1 quart heavy cream
1 cup sugar, split into three 1/3 cups
4 large eggs
1 tablespoon vanilla bean paste

Preheat oven to 300 degrees. Pour heavy cream into heavy saucepan and whisk in 1/3 cup sugar. Turn on heat to medium high. Crack eggs into a large glass-pouring cup (at least two quarts). Whisk in 1/3 cup sugar into eggs. Whisk cream until steaming but NOT boiling. *Gradually* whisk hot cream mixture into the egg mixture. Whisk in vanilla bean paste. Place shallow ramekins in large metal pan. Pour crème mixture into shallow ramekins (I use 6 ounce and even have very small 2 ounce ramekins for "tastes" of dessert). Pour hot water ½ way up outside of ramekin dishes. Gently place in oven. Bake at 300 degrees for 60 minutes. Cool for 15 minutes in water bath. Remove and place on granite to cool or refrigerate. Sprinkle with remaining sugar and torch with kitchen torch until top is caramelized.

Over 30 years ago, a journey of 30,000 miles began for a teenage runner trying to find meaning on this planet. Along the way, this is what she discovered.

CONTENTS

1

First Step

A journey of a thousand miles must begin with a single step.
~Lao Tzu

Baby we were born to run.
~Bruce Springsteen

I was sixteen years of age in December 1981, and snow was falling outside the school bus as I- trying to make a decision- stood at the white line just inside the folding door. Unbeknownst to me, that decision would affect me for the rest of my life.

Our school was sponsoring its annual "Trot for Tots", a run from Children's Hospital in Pittsburgh to our high school in Irwin, Pennsylvania, to raise money for the Marine Corps Reserve toy drive.

It was the previous year, when I was in eleventh grade when my trim trigonometry teacher, a Marine Corps reservist, first presented the run for Toys for Tots. He told us about kids who received toys on Christmas morning who would not normally have any. I yearned to participate in something positive, but I was a hurdler, jumper, and sprinter on the track team; I was not particularly proficient at any of my events, and was only running a maximum of five miles. But after a teachers' strike resulted in weeks of idleness until the first full week of school commenced in November—as well as many negative ramifications for the student body, myself included—this confused senior started dreaming.

1

Participants found sponsors to pledge a certain amount of money for each mile completed. The bus would drive all runners to Pittsburgh Children's Hospital that was approximately twenty-five miles from our school. Those who thought they could complete the distance would be dropped off there. Then there would be drop-off points every five miles until all participants were on their way.

Although I had participated on the track team since my freshman year, my longest race was the 110-yard hurdles. (Yes, it was that long ago that our races were measured in yards instead of meters.) Suffice to say that no one considered me a long-distance runner, and prior to the Trot for Tots, I had only recently began consistently running—what was for me—longer distances such as two or three miles.

Finding sponsors was easy. I think everyone who cared about me was simply excited to see me participating in life, so I had many pledges.

My goal was five miles—a goal most considered a bit lofty, and my opinion tended to equate with theirs. That is, until we reached the hospital and the music on the bus blasted Jackson Browne's "Running on Empty", and the theme from the newly released movie Chariots of Fire. I started to calculate how much more money I could raise if I departed at the ten-mile marker.

Everyone on the bus had experience with long distances. Everyone, that is but me. When we reached that hospital in the downtown Pittsburgh, snowflakes were falling. The speakers pumped Bruce Springsteen's "Born to Run." The atmosphere was electrifying.

It seemed like all the boys on the cross-country team were like horses straining to get out of the starting gate. As they took off, the rest of us on the bus were clapping wildly. As we pulled away, I started asking the cross-country girls when they were getting off the bus. Hardly any said they were departing at the twenty-mile marker.

Two of the girls, who were long-distance runners on our track team, said they were getting off at fifteen miles. "Come on, run with us," they suggested. My mind swirled with the possibility. Could it be possible? We were in old gray sweats and had pathetic shoes. Thankfully, we didn't know about Gore-Tex, Under-Armour, or high-tech shoes. The amount I could raise if I achieved this distance was considerably more substantial than I had anticipated. I told them I wanted to come with them. They were extraordinarily excited and *encouraging. More likely, though, it was incredulity that a sprinter could even conceive of such a notion.*

We were approaching the drop-off point, and I had to decide. My initial excitement began to turn to fear and anxiety. *What was I thinking? This is crazy. Stick to the plan. No one will ever know that you were considering this and didn't do it.* I stood up. Those who were planning to remain for the ten and five-mile drop-offs looked surprised, and started to cheer. The other runners had departed the bus.

Standing at that white line on the bus may just as well have been the precipice of a cliff. Time stood still. Then, I propelled myself forward down the steps with Bruce Springsteen singing in my head so I wouldn't lose my nerve, and before I knew it, the adrenaline had kicked in and we were running.

The first five miles were relatively easy, but the next five saw us struggling. Because we were thirsty and there were no refreshment stations along the way, we stopped at the only open business in the middle of one of the steel neighborhoods—a bar—and ducked inside. The looks of surprise on the men's faces were evident as they turned their attention from the television and their beers as three motley, sweaty girls asked for a drink of water.

Somehow, while we took turns using the restroom, the story of what we were doing was revealed to the patrons. I wanted nothing more than to stay in the warmth, but we started giggling at the slurred, "keep going girls" as glasses were raised.

It didn't take long for my lack of endurance training to show, so I told the others to go ahead. By the last five miles, my gait felt more like a trudge on the mostly-desolate Route 993. A hitchhiker held up his thumb on the other side of the road. While I didn't sense I was in danger, I knew that if he decided to chase me, I was already running as fast as I could muster.

Shortly thereafter, my father came driving up along my side of the road from out of nowhere honking his horn and cheering as loudly as he could.

He told me that I just had about a mile to go before the big hill up ahead and I was almost there. Although I desperately wanted to jump in his car, I just kept going. He turned the car around to head back to the high school, picking up the hitchhiker on the way, honking his horn, and pumping his fist out the window as he went by me. I laughed at the thought of my mother being furious at him for giving a ride to the stranger, and at my own stupidity for not hitching a ride myself.

However, it was just the encouragement needed for me to finish the race.

When I made it back, I was numb from either the pain or the cold. But even more so, I was numb from the fact that I had won a pair of good running shoes for the amount of money I had raised.

Those New Balance shoes changed my life. Kids at school were incredulous when it was announced on the loudspeaker the following Monday morning. None of that mattered. The path of my life had become a runner's, but it all came down to a line on a school bus, a dash of Bruce Springsteen, and a single step.

Humanity is linked by a common instinctual desire that crosses cultural, social, political and religious boundaries. From infancy, there are physical and emotional needs that must be met, and then there are some that should be met. There is just one desire, however, that most healthy babies will fulfill in their own time. They pull themselves up, take a first step, toddle and fall, and eventually walk on their own. When they do, they will try to, well, *accelerate.*

Truly, have you seen a baby take that first monumental step, and then sit down for months on end, basking in the achievement without relishing to string as many of those steps together as quickly as possible?

John Ortberg, a pastor from Menlo Park Presbyterian Church in California, wrote an entire book, *If You Want to Walk on Water, You Have to Get Out of the Boat,* about eight verses from the fourteenth chapter of the gospel of Matthew where Peter ventures out of the safety of a vessel into waves towards Jesus.

Perhaps because the expression, "walk on water," is used in speech, most people know this story well, even if they haven't heard it on a Sunday morning in church. Jesus is walking on water and Peter attempts to walk toward Him, notices the strong wind and begins to sink. Each insightful exploration in Ortberg's book is a revelation in and of itself, but what is especially notable in his assessment of Peter is that it reveals Peter as a great success story for having simply gotten out of the boat.

Think about it. Even famous artists throughout history usually depict Peter in his act of failure, being submerged by the water, rescued by Jesus. Even without traveling, the images are familiar, such as *Navicella*, the mosaic in St. Peter's Basilica in Vatican City by Giotta. In this mosaic, Peter is already holding onto the hand of Jesus, having already been saved by the hero of the story. So consider Peter's success. *He* was the one who left the boat. *He* was the one who risked the opportunity of a lifetime.

The *other* disciples on the other hand, the ones who chose to stay in the boat, were the real failures in the passage.

Ortberg writes regarding the other disciples, *"They understood the cost of getting out of the boat. They were very much aware of the pain of potential failure, embarrassment, inadequacy, criticism, and perhaps even loss of life."* He goes on to say, *"But what they were not so aware of was another price – the cost of staying in the boat."*

We label those who are watching life go by from a Barcalounger "couch potatoes," but Ortberg calls them "boat potatoes."

What would your life look like with one single step? In some ways, that's exactly how my journey began—with a single step down a school bus stair at the age of sixteen. Then I stepped down again, unknowingly beginning a journey that is still being defined to this day. Thanks, Bruce Springsteen.

Pondering for the Road

What is it that first step you feel called to take? If you are sure the timing is right, whether a career change, an exercise program, starting a new relationship, fixing an old relationship, eating healthier? Seize the day! If you can't motivate yourself to move those little toes past the little white line, perhaps there's someone you trust to give you a little push.

My Prayer for You

My prayer for you today is that you can be relieved of the burden of wondering what it feels like to take that step, regardless of the outcome.

Sustenance for the Road

In his heart a man plans his course, but the LORD determines his steps. Proverbs 16:9

How do you want to go forward?

_____

_____

_____

Do you have a story regarding the first step?
Tell it at www.whatilearnedwhilerunning.com

2

Prayer, Answered and Unanswered

Therefore I tell you, whatever you ask for in prayer,
believe you have received it, and it will be yours.
Mark 11:24

Sometimes, I thank God for unanswered prayer.
~Garth Brooks

It was late summer of 1982, and the song "Tainted Love" by Soft Cell was playing loudly on the radio of my parents' Volkswagen Rabbit as I pulled into the high school parking lot to run the cross-country course. Ever since the Trot for Tots, the mileage of my runs has been slowly and consistently increasing. As the song finished, and I turned off the car to silence, I once again yearned to be able to listen to music while running. Specifically, I was yearning for a Sony Walkman.

Like all students getting ready to head to college, I had been purchasing items for my dorm room at Penn State, such as bedding and toiletries. To say my budget from working as a summer janitor cleaning the elementary school was limited would be an overstatement. As nice as it would be to own a Sony Walkman, at one hundred dollars, it was just too expensive. Still, I wanted one.

When my friend brought two headsets for us to run together and listen to music, the time just seemed to fly by, and there was just so much good music.

I prayed that perhaps someone would give one to me as a graduation present, so that I could use it at college.

That didn't happen, so in the meantime, I continued to run without a Walkman. Sometimes I prayed the rosary, and sometimes I recited in my mind the sine and cosine of all the angles from my trigonometry class. Yes, thanks to Mr. Shirley, I knew that both the sine and cosine of forty-five degrees are the square root of two over two, and a few miles could go by as I envisioned all 360 degrees in my mind. It was a meaningless talent except that my mind was unencumbered with the distance that passed by so quickly, and then it was quite useful.

I arrived at college Walkman-less. Of course I saw all the kids on campus wearing theirs and I, thinking it would improve my quality of life, still wanted one, especially while running. Interestingly enough, I didn't envy those who were in possession of my coveted device.

So months went by. On home football game days, I jogged in the morning, and laughed and waved when I heard the Fiji fraternity brothers yelling to me from the parking lot of my two older brothers' fraternity.

Tuning into all the sounds around me, I heard the crunch of fall leaves beneath my feet, and the soft start of snowfall on the leaves that had yet to fall. Fluffy big flakes melted instantly on my tongue. Dogs barking in the distance were easy to discern as well as those close enough to warrant stopping and holding my hand out, palm up in peace.

The quiet of glistening deep snow soon gave way to the music of robins, woodpeckers and mourning doves in springtime. Besides hearing the proximity of other runners coming up behind me, my other senses were heightened as well, and I felt the wind, as it could not decide if it wanted to leave winter behind. Before the distant thunder foretells it will rain, I have already tasted the raindrops on my lips. And, if the smell of hyacinths or freshly mowed grass wasn't tantalizing enough after a long Pennsylvania winter, the scent of neighborhood barbecue grills certainly was.

Before long, I found myself looking forward to leaving the noise of lecture halls, cafeterias and dormitories. Loops around the Blue and White Golf Courses revealed an evening glow as the setting sun gave way to twilight. Mornings were equally exquisite with the morning mist rising from fields surrounding Beaver Stadium, Mount Nittany in the distance. There was always something breathtaking to see, hear, smell, taste and touch. Beauty that could stop me in my tracks. My Walkman-less life was alive with an intimacy with God's creation and sometimes, even for a fleeting moment, I am sure God revealed Himself as well.

The time came when I could have bought the coveted item of my prayers, but I opted against doing so. This is not to say that running to music is in any way a wrong thing to do. In fact, there is research to suggest that performance is enhanced when exercising to upbeat songs. * Even though I desired it, I didn't think it was wrong to do so, and occasionally borrowed headphones to run.

However, the sixth chapter of the gospel of Matthew says, "Do not store up for yourselves treasure on earth, where moth and rust destroy... For where your treasure is, there your heart will be also." Evaluating where our treasure is *does* tell us where our heart is.

Recently, there was an item in my home that my four sons fought over for possession. This coveted treasure wasn't a video game, piece of sports equipment, or a computer, but they would race for "first dibs" on it. Ironically, given my history regarding the Sony Walkman, it wasn't even their phones. No, the item of contention was dryer lint. Clothing dryer lint. When the sound was heard of the completed dryer, chaos would ensue as the boys clamored to be the first to pull out the screen to claim their ball of lint.

No, it was not an unusual hoarding ritual, but even if it was, it was an unusual battle to referee. To say the dryer is going very frequently when you are raising four boys on a farm is an understatement. Even if blankets and sheets are hung outside to dry, there is no way *not* to use the dryer for endless football and baseball gear, even if the jerseys must be hung to dry (who chose white baseball pants?), wrestling gear, jeans, and mismatched socks. Thus, we have a lot of lint, enough to go around. Why were my sons knocking each other down, racing to the dryer to be the first to the lint screen? Certainly not to fold clothing and put it away. Two reasons: birds and fire.

The first reason was because a birdwatcher that works with my husband shared that if you place lint in an empty net bag, the type in which clementines, potatoes, or onions are sold, and then hang the bag from a tree, birds would use the lint to pad their nests.** Secondly, during a winter survival snowshoe course at our middle school, the students were taught one of the best items to have to start a fire is lint.

As you can imagine, the boys were willing to test the fire theory frequently and successfully, whether in the outside bonfire pit, or in the fireplace. Although not a matter of survival, the many Ziploc bags of lint helped when the electricity went out and a morning chore was to rekindle a fire that seemed to have exhausted itself from the night before. Soon thereafter, we saw the first nest of baby robins cozy in their home of twigs softened with denim lint, and my first thought was that they would be fighting over dryer lint for the rest of their lives. Thankfully, they all went on to their next heartfelt desires such as shooting their first turkey, being the first to jump in the neighbors' pond for the summer, getting new chicks (the kind that lay eggs), etc.

According to the world's standards, prayers are either answered which is good, or unanswered, which is bad, and thus reflective of a God that does not provide. Oswald Chambers challenged that notion in the renowned devotional, *My Utmost for His Highest.* In First Thessalonians 5:17, the verse "Pray without ceasing," prompted Chambers to give this commentary.

"We think rightly or wrongly about prayer according to the conception we have in our minds of prayer. If we think of prayer as the breath in our lungs and the blood from our hearts, we think rightly...

...do we think of the times when God does not seem to have answered prayer? 'Every one that asketh receiveth.' We say-"But...,but..." God answers prayer in the best way, not sometimes, but every *time, although the immediate manifestation of the answer in the domain in which we want it may not always follow."*

So while I thought my prayer was to have a Sony Walkman, my real prayer was to be able to continue to enjoy running longer distances, a prayer that was answered in the best possible way, without becoming dependent upon a device. Because my senses were allowed, unencumbered, to be attentive to the world around me, my life as a runner was immensely blessed, and the lesson of what I thought was unanswered prayer became a precious gift that became part of the journey.

So, many years after that Walkman-less freshman year, I experienced what would be my last and final pregnancy—with twins, hoping with a heart's desire that they would be girls (after four boys-need I say more?). It was not to be as I ended up miscarrying, which was a heartbreaking time for me, especially because I felt I had to internalize so much of my feelings for my sons' sake and because our lives were just so busy with the end of a large stressful construction project, amongst our normal demands.

Within a few years, a set of precious twin girls came into our lives, bringing unspeakable joy to my life. Accompanying them to summer camp one year, I realized that if my own babies had survived, there would have been no time to invest in these girls' lives, no long talks about the books we are reading, no winter sale shopping excursions for cute coats, no laugh-so-hard-the-chair-breaks games of 'spoons'. It was then that the realization came to me that my prayer was for twin girls not *daughters*.

Tears of grief transformed to tears of joy with *answered* prayer.

Pondering for the Road

What are you praying for at this time? Could you consider this prayer going "unanswered" and rephrasing your prayer and allowing it to be answered in another way—like my twin girls?

My Prayer for You

If God does not grant you what you desire and pray for, my prayer is that He will either remove the desire from your heart, or fulfill that desire in another way.

Sustenance for the Road

Psalm 37:4 says Delight yourself in the Lord and he will give you the desires of your heart

How do you want to go forward?

_____

_____

_____

Tell your story regarding answered prayer at
whatilearnedwhilerunning.com

*This is something to which I can attest, having played "Bad Moon Rising" by Credence Clearwater Revival in my mind to increase my pace in many Army Physical Training Tests in college.

**Recently, I learned that if you use laundry detergent with harsh chemicals and strong fragrances, that the lint can be harmful for birds.

Colleen Tretter

3

RUN YOUR OWN RACE

You were running a good race. Who cut in on you…?
Galatians 5:7

And I saw that all labor and all achievement
spring from man's envy of his neighbor. This too
is meaningless, a chasing after the wind.
Ecclesiastes 4:4

Now famous for her work with St. Jude's Children's Hospital, Marlo Thomas was renowned to the baby boomer generation for her portrayal as Ann Marie in the hit television series "That Girl" from the late 1960s and early 1970s. In her book, *The Right Words At The Right Time,* Thomas tells the story of how her famous father gave her a gift that taught her a most precious lesson as she too, entered show business.

Her father, Danny Thomas, once said to her, "*I raised you to be a thoroughbred. When thoroughbreds run, they wear blinders to keep their eyes focused straight ahead with no distractions, no other horses. They hear the crowd but they don't listen. They just run their own race. That's what you have to do. Don't listen to anyone comparing you to me or to anyone else. You just run your own race.*"

With the exception of "I love you," these may just be the some of the best words any father has said to any daughter. If all children were encouraged to run their own race, how different the world might look.

The energy expended on striving to compare one's life to others could be directed more purposefully. But Mr. Thomas took it one step further.

He made his point crystal clear as Ms. Thomas recounts,

The next night as the crowd filed into the theater, the stage manager knocked on my dressing room door and handed me a white box with a red ribbon. I opened it up and inside was a pair of old horse blinders with a little note that read, "Run your own race, Baby."

How important is it to run one's own race, without giving way to comparisons and contrasts, whether in how one looks, how one performs or what one has? Well, if *not* running one's own race leads to the so-called green-eyed monster of jealousy, then it is crucially important. According to Proverbs 14:30, *a heart at peace gives life to the body, but envy rots the bones.* When Jesus was teaching the legalistic Pharisees about their inner hearts in the seventh chapter of the gospel of Mark, he lumped envy in with theft, murder, adultery, and greed.

Growing up, my favorite book was *The Sneetches* by Dr. Seuss. Although we had books all over our house, I adored that one the most. I loved reading about the Plain-Belly Sneetches getting their stars after they were treated so terribly by the Star-Belly Sneetches. The illustration of Sylvester McMonkey McBean's machine as he charged Sneetches for stars on, then stars off, fascinated me.

Did reading about the Sneetches change my perspective about envying others? Perhaps. More likely the reason was having been raised in a family of six children as well as whatever needy individual we would bring home to our chaotic but fun open-door household. It taught me to appreciate those with stars and those without, and to never yearn to run through McBean's machine. In other words, it taught me to run my own race before I knew what that meant.

Many things cut in on us in our own races. External pressures such as a health crisis, unemployment, a failed relationship, and financial struggles, can sabotage our direction and focus. Worse yet, judgment from others or judgment from our own selves can be the real crippler.

One of my favorite running quotes is from *Chariots of Fire,* the fact-based 1981 Academy Award winner for best motion picture.

"I believe that God made me for a purpose... But He also made me fast, and when I run I feel His pleasure. To give it up would be to hold Him in contempt."

The quote is attributed to Eric Liddell, the Christian Scot whose deep faith gives him his purpose, however he never actually said these words; Colin Welland, writer of the screenplay, wrote them, beautiful words that are inspirational even thirty years after the movie was released.

Another famous historical runner who achieved one of the most remarkable accomplishments in sports history was when British athlete, Roger Bannister, broke the elusive 4-minute mile in 1954, six-tenths of a second under the historic barrier. Lauded with accolades, including a knighthood in his native England, his accomplishment on the track isn't what he considers his greatest in life. Rather his career as a physician practicing neurology for many years after that historical day is the achievement that garnered his greatest contentment.

Roger Banister ran his own race and allowed no one to cut in on him. Not pride, arrogance, or a lifetime of resting on his laurels. Being the first to break the four-minute mile mark is epic, akin to being the first to climb Mount Everest or walk on the moon. Even if people do recall Edmund Hillary and Neil Armstrong more readily, Roger Banister is in their league. Others may achieve it, but no one else can say they were the first to do it. Still, years later, Bannister never forgot to give accolades to the two pace makers who helped him, Chris Brasher and Chris Chataway.

Conversely, one of the most heartbreaking races to hear about happened in 1986 when college athlete Kathy Ormsby of North Carolina State, a collegiate record-holder in the women's 10,000-meter race, was running in the NCAA outdoor track and field championships at Indiana University Track. For the first 6,500 meters, she was in the top four, well ahead of the rest of the field, but she was struggling and fell behind the other runners. Everyone in the stadium, including her family members, watched as she ran off the track, and out of the stadium. Before anyone could find her, she ran to a nearby bridge over the White River and jumped, landing in weeds rather than the water.

Surviving the jump but sustaining a severe spinal cord injury, Ormsby gave her first interview later that year when she was adjusting to life with paralysis from the waist down, citing the perfectionism that plagued her career and something in her that "just snapped. Perhaps those around her really tried to alleviate her fear of failure, but somehow or another she was not content to run her own race if it meant her performance was anything but exceptional.

So often the battle is waged in our own minds, and we lose our focus. Where can we reclaim our focus? The entire verse of Galatians 5:7 says: *You were running a good race. Who cut in on you and kept you from obeying the truth?*

Obeying what truth? The Apostle Paul says that it is for freedom that Christ has set us free. Freedom. Not for following legalistic rules, or for the slavery of trying to be justified by what we do right or what we don't do wrong. This is untruth that allows us to fall away from grace. No one is immune to the danger. In verse six, he makes clear what truly matters: *The only thing that counts is faith expressing itself through love.* But how? Verse thirteen tells us how our freedom should be used. "*Serve one another in love.*"

People serve one another in love in many different ways. In our community, there is a residential summer camp for children and adults with mental and developmental disabilities called Camp PARC (People Always Responding with Compassion). In existence for more than half a century, most of those years have involved Ted and Judy Risch. Now serving at the helm of the organization, the Rischs express their faith through love for the campers year after year. They have been instrumental in creating an opportunity for many, many children, teenagers and adults to also serve one another in love.

Volunteers such as junior counselors, typically teenagers, are responsible for the campers nearly the entire week. Also included in the army of volunteers serving one another in love are kitchen staffs that cook and happily present food everyone enjoys. It would be remiss of me to not testify that the blessing of being able to serve has been extended to me as well, because the medical need of the camp is great. So, running around as the camp nurse allows me to see and experience the ineffable joy of campers and volunteers alike.

Evaluating what might be thwarting us from serving others is a healthy exercise. Allowing our race to be "cut in on" is just what the enemy desires, so that we can't experience freedom, or allowing our faith to be expressed through love. Anything that immobilizes, anything that paralyzes, anything that stops us from a life of faith expressing itself through love is NOT from God. It is a lie from the darkest forces of the universe. Staying in motion requires the connectivity to the power of all that is good, all that is true, all that is lovely, all that is worthy, and all that is our Sovereign God. There are many forces that can unbalance us, even good ones, such as loved ones with the best of intentions for our lives, or valid causes that interrupt our momentum by vying for our time.

Other times, *we* are the unbalanced force, as I learned in 1985 while running with my fiancée, Jim.

We were running together through the streets of my hometown. Although we had known each other for less than a year, we were taking a leap of faith and entering into the sacrament of marriage at Christmastime. Our cadre Captain, Michael Madonna, had taken us aside and inquired if we were considering the possibility of a future together. We told him we had. He advised us that with Jim already having been commissioned in the U.S. Army, and my impending paperwork for the same just after the New Year in 1986, we had better make a commitment. We had spent the summer apart while I was a cadet nurse at Walter Reed Army Medical Center, and were apart again as he was in school in New York and I was back for my last semester at Hershey, Pennsylvania.

During weekends when we could spend time together, Jim's faster pace was distinctly noticeable. Every now and then my competitive streak would get the best of me, and I would try to finish our course first, and then he would accelerate. It frustrated me immensely if he beat me at the end.

On this day when it was evident he would again be victorious, I saw a dead snake on the ground, and since he didn't seem to have seen it, I bent down to pick it up and put it in the pocket of my sweatshirt. He was waiting for me, trotting slowly near our completion point, and I slowed and started walking, and said, "Yes, you smoked me again," as I reached into my pocket, acted surprised and said, "What's this? AAAAAAHHHG!!!" I yelled, and I threw it at him!

Unbeknownst to me, he had a snake phobia, like Indiana Jones Raiders of the Lost Ark snake phobia. Ever since one of the snakes he caught as a child coiled up and bit him, he had an unsettled fear of them, but it was one of the things in our relatively short courtship that he failed to share.

In my defense, this is a man who completed Army Airborne (parachuting out of airplanes) and Air Assault (parachuting out of helicopters) Schools, and an avid hunter and outdoorsman, so it didn't occur to me that he had fears. So when this snake came flailing at him in the air, he obviously didn't know that it was dead, and he jumped about two feet in the air thrashing his arms and legs wildly. Even when he was able to discern that it was not actually a live snake, he nearly fainted! He was pale and sweating profusely, but not from the run, I assure you.

I was the unbalanced force that acted upon his speed and direction. After that, we made it a point to try to tell each other every pertinent thing the other should know before our wedding. Thankfully, he still married me, and nearly thirty years later, our vows stand.

Don't let anyone or anything cut in on you. Don't be the force that cuts in on someone else. And don't toss dead snakes around. Run your own race.

Pondering for the Road

Is something, someone, or your own judgment "cutting in on you" in your race? Discern which one it is, and then meditate how to thwart this influence.

My Prayer for You

That you may have blinders on your eyes that you may see straight ahead the race marked out for you! Yours is a glorious path that God intended for you and you alone. No one else can "run" your race for you. It is yours, and I pray that you embrace it as it is, that you resist anything or anyone not of God that cuts in on you, and that you cross the finish line triumphant!

Sustenance for the Road

Therefore, there is now no condemnation for those who are in Christ Jesus, because through Christ Jesus the law of the Spirit of life set me free from the law of sin and death. Romans 8:1

How do you want to go forward?

_____

_____

_____

Have a story about running your own race? Tell it at whatilearnedwhilerunning.com.

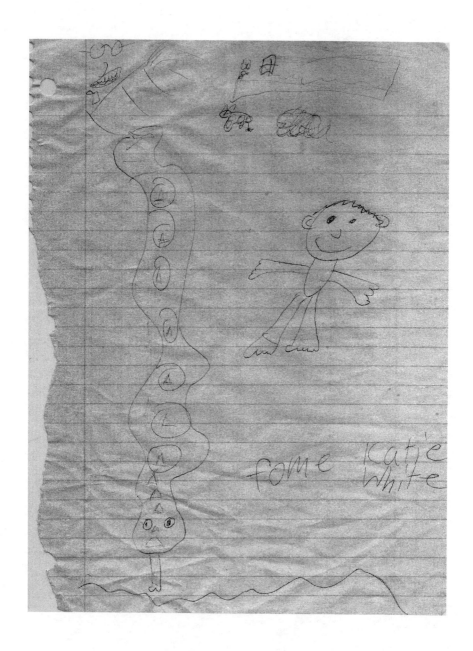

In 1998, we brought our son, Paul, home from Hawaii to the farm to celebrate his first birthday with family and friends. Our closest friends from college, Tim and Susan White, allowed their three daughters to stay with us while they attended a conference in California. On one of the days, Jim brought all the kids on a hike. They encountered a snake. (Please take note that this is thirteen years after my snake story). Kathleen "Katie" White and her sisters returned to tell me how high Uncle Jim jumped in the air when they came across a snake. Katie was convinced I didn't understand HOW HIGH as she lifted her little hand as high as it would go, so she made me a drawing. Note the ground. Today she is a graduate of Temple University with a degree in Art and works in Philadelphia. Much of her work as ktwhite brings me great joy, but none quite like her work as a little girl!

4

Running Will Take Care of You, If You Take Care of Your Feet.

…you also should wash one another's feet.
Jesus to his disciples as told in the Gospel of John 13:14

Life is too short to wear tight shoes.
~Quote on journal, author unknown

In our present culture, because of ubiquitous nail salons in malls, spas and schools of cosmetology, even young girls have manicures and pedicures. Not so in "ancient times," as my sons call my younger days. Well into my thirties when I finally had my first pedicure, I could not believe what I had been missing. If heaven existed for feet alone, it would begin in a swirling pedicure tub.

Each phase of my first pedicure was even better than the previous one, from soaking in a warm basin of water, to the mint foot scrub. Then came the pumice treatment. Quietly, the technician inquired, "Are you a runner?" I told her that, why yes I was and inquired as to what gave it away.

Ever since an old boyfriend told me we had matching calf muscles (and his, quite frankly, were unattractive), it just became one of the many things about which I was self-conscious. Was she going to say my legs were ugly? So, when the aesthetician exclaimed, "Your feet are a mess!" I was somewhat relieved. Callouses and rough, dry skin do have a way of piling up over thirty years.

Running will take care of you...

So how will running take care of you? Well, it is the antidote for just about whatever ails you. One of the most widely touted benefits is that running not only increases the release of powerful endorphins, but also the "feel good" chemical, serotonin, while decreasing the negative stress chemical, cortisol.

In the 2001 movie, *Legally Blonde*, Elle Woods (played by Reese Witherspoon) is a beautiful blonde Harvard Law School student. She is an intern on the legal defense team of a wealthy woman who is accused of murdering her elderly husband. When Elle realizes that this defendant is her older sorority sister and renowned fitness magnate, Brooke Taylor, Elle comes to her defense. The rest of the legal team consists mostly of men who believe the wealthy client is guilty. In a sweet perky voice, Elle sums up her reasoning for her fitness idol's innocence:

"I just don't think Brooke could have done this. Exercise gives you endorphins. Endorphins make you happy. Happy people just don't shoot their husbands... They just don't!"

In more recent years, the benefit of running reducing the stress chemical, cortisol, has been emphasized. Cortisol has been found to be so detrimental that in Psychology Today, writer Chris Bergland, entitled it "Public Enemy No. 1," when chronically exposed to it.

In a classic "fight or flight" situation, cortisol release is a positive response, such as escaping from a building on fire. However, in sustained situations, over long periods of time, such as high stress occupations, or prolonged traumas, it has been shown to cause increased fat deposit around vital organs. Additionally, it has been linked to elevated blood pressure, hindered memory, as well as less serious maladies.

Medical research has proven that running can help in the prevention and treatment of cardiovascular disease, high blood pressure, diabetes, and depression. Exercise, as long as it is not performed just prior to bedtime, aids in the overall improvement of sleep. Exercise performed when drowsy has been found to create alertness. There are reports of improved sexual health in those who are exercising regularly, whether from an innate sense of wellbeing, or increased contentment with self-image.

Moreover, because running is a weight-bearing activity, it strengthens bones, while exercises such as swimming and biking cannot make that claim. But did you know that recent research shows cancer patients tolerate chemo and radiation better with exercise? Or that a study published by the Centers for Disease Control and Prevention shows that kids who exercise have better grades than sedentary peers?

Then there is the obvious obesity epidemic impacting our nation. Look at old photographs. It is surprisingly shocking that so few obese people are visible. It was distinctly noticeable when pictures recently emerged from the parade route of John F. Kennedy's infamous motorcade for example, that obesity is obviously just recently representative of our current population. One projection by Trust for America's Health and the Robert Wood Johnson Foundation predicts that by 2030 over 50 percent of the population in most states will be obese.

Whatever ails you, running or exercise is good medicine, which is not to say that you won't still need your medicine. Perhaps you will need less, as is widely touted in media exposure of contestants on the reality show *The Biggest Loser*.

In the movie, *My Big Fat Greek Wedding*, the main character, Toula, says of her father, who is frequently seen with a bottle of Windex that he sprays prolifically, "My dad believes in two things. That Greeks should educate non-Greeks about being Greek, and any ailment from psoriasis to poison ivy could be cured with Windex."

So, in the *My Big Fat Greek Wedding* of life, running is the Windex. It is the cure to almost any malady.

Furthermore, there are few *negative* addictive behaviors that can be done while running. You seldom see runners smoking cigarettes or compulsively overeating, at least while they're running.

The only addictive behavior where running is not beneficial is if your addiction happens to be running. Make no mistake about it; it can be as detrimental as a drug addiction. Indeed, it is a drug addiction; the chemicals just happen to be supplied by one's own body. What makes one runner "hooked" beyond healthy and another runner indifferent is probably the same reason some people smoke and get addicted to cigarettes while others are unaffected.

There was a time in my teens when running was my life. It seemed my happiness revolved around it, and yet I was still miserable. Every runner should ask the question, "Do I live to run or do I run to live?" We'll visit this later, but ask yourself the question, "Is it your god?"

In 1990, one of the first articles on the subject of running addiction appeared in the *Journal of Sports Medicine and Physical Fitness*. The authors, Carol Chapman and John DeCastro, reported on a senior thesis study that evaluated runners' responses to a running addiction scale, RAS, as well as a differentiation between a commitment to running versus an evaluable addiction.

Based on my own personal experience and from observations of other runners who seem to be in the throes of addiction, here is a questionnaire to visit. The following questions, adapted from many "addictive questionnaires" can give insight as to which side of the track, so to speak, a runner may fall. While not a scientific quiz, it can be enlightening. Believe me, there was a time when I could answer "yes" to more than a few questions, so if the questions make you squirm or touch a nerve, my empathy is with you. However, this may reveal something that is hindering a more abundant life. Take a breath and answer as truthfully as possible. Better yet, ask a friend or significant other what they think your answers should be.

1. My family and friends complain about my running.
2. People (family, friends, co-workers, etc.) just don't understand my running.
3. I would rather be running than at most social gatherings.
4. I have missed events that are important to people close to me because I was running.
5. I feel guilty if I miss a run.
6. I have run with injuries and pain.
7. I have run against the advice of a physician.
8. I have run when conditions/weather were adverse: fog, darkness, lightning, snowstorm, and icy roads.
9. My free time and money is spent on participating in races regularly.
10. Running is my life.
11. I have regularly neglected household chores/responsibilities to run (ha ha! I have regularly neglected household chores to do anything!

It's not wrong to want to stay in shape, but I know of a dad who missed his child's sporting event because of his own running priority. Now, you may justify that as perfectly reasonable. However, that justification, and an uncomfortable response evoked by these statements may just be shedding light on an addiction that is prohibiting you from enjoying running to its fullest, because if it isn't improving the quality of your life, enhancing your relationships, promoting your health and well-being, then what good is it?

Thankfully, for no specific reason, and through a transition that was not particularly defined, I came out to the other side fairly quickly to where running only enhanced the quality of my life, which continues to this day.

If you take care of your feet...

And how you do that, primarily is investing in the best shoes your feet require. Most sports require equipment that can be expensive such as helmets, kneepads, racquets, bicycles, and the like. Or the recreation requires having access to a specific facility such as a swimming pool, or ice skating rink, or is dependent upon other individuals to participate, such as tennis and basketball (beyond just shooting practice). Even sports with the dubious distinction of actually being sports, such as golf, or bowling, require costly gear.

For the casual runner, it almost doesn't matter how you run. Remember Phoebe in the television series *Friends*? Rachel is embarrassed to run with her in Central Park because Phoebe's arms and legs flail. At first, the empathy sits with Rachel, until Phoebe explains that she runs with the pure bliss of childhood and doesn't care what others think. Suddenly Rachel, too, wants to experience the unhindered joy. The episode ends with the two of them flailing together through Central Park.

Quite a few endeavors should not be undertaken without proper instruction and guidance. (Just kidding about the golf thing. Calm down, golfers!) The beautiful thing about running is that just about everyone on the planet has done it at some point in life. So if you don't think you're a runner, at one time you most assuredly were!

What does matter, however, is proper footwear and decent socks. You wouldn't play basketball in cleats or soccer in basketball shoes, so under no circumstances (with the exception of escaping a criminal, and yes, statistics show running away is your best option even if the criminal has a gun) should you attempt to run any significant distance in anything except a shoe built for running. True, proper shoes can be pricey, but this is one area where there should be no skimping.

Think of it another way. The outlay of money is just for shoes – not on a gym membership, equipment, or special clothing, because it really doesn't matter what you wear (unless of course you are running at night and then you should most definitely have reflective gear). Moreover, if you experience pain because of improper footwear, not only are you less likely to continue to achieve your goals, but also can actually injure yourself.

Where to begin? Certainly copious availability of shoes in large sporting good stores is an option. But if you are a novice, you really want someone with expertise who can help you—not just a college kid filling in a time slot—unless that employee is a knowledgeable runner.

Finding out what type of foot you have is the very first thing to do. Wetting your foot and stepping on a piece of paper very easily accomplishes this. You will be able to ascertain if you have a high arch, flat foot, etc. Next, do you pronate or supinate (lean heavily on the inside or outside of your foot)? Find a pair of shoes you wear frequently and look at the back of them at eye level. If they are more worn on the insides, you pronate. Conversely, if the outside edges reveal more wear, you supinate. You will need to find a shoe that provides stability to compensate for your natural step.

If the soles are even, you have a stable foot. Regardless, there are other factors that you will need to address such as cushioning and the amount of toe room you need. There are companies with excellent resources. You can speak with specialists regarding these and other issues, and some companies will even permit you to order and try out shoes indoors, and allow you to return them as long as you don't wear them outdoors. Once you find shoes that work, buy a second pair if possible. Many runners firmly believe that by alternating shoes on consecutive runs (for example, running one run in your red shoes, and the next in your blue), those two pairs of shoes could last eighteen months whereas two pairs, each worn until they were no longer usable, would last only twelve months (six months each).

Lastly, proper socks are essential for maximum comfort. By trial and error, one can easily determine the qualities preferred in athletic socks such as cushioning, breathability, or blister reducing.

Don't forget "one another's feet."

A few years ago, during a medical mission trip to Haiti, the pastor highlighted this message from the thirteenth chapter of John, describing the significance of Jesus washing the disciples' feet just before the Passover Feast.

Many of us on the trip were runners, yet it wasn't safe to venture anywhere alone, not even one hundred yards unaccompanied by a "buddy." When you are blessed with the freedom of moving miles at a time, whenever or wherever you wish, a restriction such as this is palpable. One of the physicians (the "buffest guy in the county" according to my oldest son) would work out in place, by jumping and climbing stairs.

The biblical passage tells of Simon Peter saying to Jesus, "No, you shall never wash my feet." Most everyone has heard the response of Jesus at one time or another, "Unless I wash you, you have no part with me."

While the message of being humble enough to serve others is the primary lesson to be learned, especially in this narcissistic society – I believe it was called "Ego Nation" on the news recently – what seems to be more difficult for most of the people I know is Peter's problem. It seems we have become so self-sufficient in our society that we don't let ourselves be served. No, no, no, *you* will not wash *my* feet (especially without a proper pedicure).

To rally around others and provide emotional, physical, financial support is easy. Receiving it – there's the rub for some of us.

That buff doctor shared an occurrence he experienced which depicts this perfectly. When he is not on overseas mission trips, or volunteering in the local free medical clinic, or serving in his church, he trains.

Locally, there is a 70-mile trail along the Pennsylvania Laurel Mountains. Some folks hike it over a few days, camping in sites along the way. A group of lunatics came up with the brilliant idea that they should try to run it in one day.

Now, this is rough terrain. This is not like a city marathon, which is tough enough, along paved streets with cheering crowds and beautiful sights to admire along the way.

This is an isolated, nearly three-marathon distance on a trail that, even in sunny dry weather, a few miles hiking requires vigilance for participants to avoid tripping on tree roots and stones. It's a run for the elite. Not all of the elite finish.

After finishing in a state of exhaustion, cold and spent, this physician relays the story of how he cannot even bend over to remove his shoes. His wife, waiting at the finish line, gently removes the last vestiges of his grueling effort and places comfortable sandals upon his feet.

Remarkable, isn't it? An act of simple grace is embedded in our mind's eye, as a reminder how some of us must learn to receive so that others can serve.

Perhaps this scenario is elusive to you. Perhaps the narcissistic scale tips in your favor. You never think of "washing others' feet," and wouldn't even know where to begin to help someone else. A woman I have come to care deeply for has been enmeshed in self-centeredness as she heals from years of addiction, having relied on American society for many basic needs such as food, housing and health care. When she told me she was helping to watch a neighbor's child, and washed all the dishes in their home, it was a sure sign that she was emerging to the other side where she could wash others' feet.

You don't need to be in ministry or a foreign mission field to wash one another's feet. All you need is what Ephesians 6:15 says you need which is this: *your feet fitted with the readiness that comes from the gospel of peace.* Are your feet fitted with readiness?

Pondering for the Road

Are you someone who readily serves, but has a difficult time receiving from others? Ask yourself if you are the type of person who needs to wash someone else's feet? Do you allow your own to be washed? Think this one out, then return to the lesson of chapter one and take the first step.

My Prayer for You

My prayer for you is that you will run to live rather than live to run, and that those who love you can readily say that it not only enhances your life, but theirs as well because of the person you are.

Sustenance for the Road

"How beautiful are the feet of those who bring good news!"

Romans 10:15

How do you want to go forward?

_____

_____

_____

Do you have a story to share regarding running taking care of you, or washing one another's feet? Share it at whatilearnedwhilerunning.com.

5

THE PRIZE

Do you not know that in a race all the runners run, but only
one gets the prize? Run in such a way as to get the prize.
Everyone who competes in the games goes into strict training.
1 Corinthians 9:24, 25

I press on towards the goal to win the prize for
which God has called me heavenward...
Philippians 3:14

Winning matters. But, on the flip side, does it really matter? Who won
the World Series two years ago? Unless your favorite team was in it, you
probably won't recall. A more significant question might be to ask the
name of the victorious team in the Super Bowl two years ago. If you are
a vigilante of sports, can you name the winner from even three years ago
since it is the most widely watched globally televised event?

In the 2011 inspirational handbook by Sam Parker, *212 the extra
degree*, the spoils of victory are made clear. The premise of the book is
that, at 211 degrees, you just have very hot water. Add one more degree
Fahrenheit, the water boils, and *"with boiling water, comes steam...and with
steam you can power a train."* Now, this book is very inspirational, but for
those of us who love to cook, Parker had us at "boiling water," and though
I shouldn't include others in my shortsightedness, my vision isn't ambitious
enough to consider powering a train. It is impressive enough to just be able

to turn what would be a clump of pasta in hot water to perfect linguini. And don't even get me started on steaming perfect Thai sticky rice! *

In the handbook, the differentiation of the "extra degree" results in the difference between reaping a prize usually associated with first place, versus second place. Quite often the slightest margin of time can mean a vast monetary divide in those prizes. An excellent example of this in the book is the following statement:

Two of auto racing's premier events are the Daytona 500 (stock car) and the Indianapolis 500 (Indy car). Each takes roughly three to three and a half hours to complete. In the 15-year period between 1996 and 2010, combining all 30 races, the winner took the checkered flag by an average margin of less than a second (0.84) and took home $1,557,914 in first place prize money. The average prize for the second place finisher was $794,191 – a difference of $763,723 – roughly half of the amount banked by the winner.

So for the victors of these races and many other competitions listed in the book, winning *matters*.

Yet, all one needs to do is to go to a local field day at an elementary school to witness the truth. Regardless of the race, a heartfelt exuberance ensues from every participant in the competition, whether in a 50-meter dash, or a relay race. Not a single youngster gimps along as if the race doesn't matter, and the prize is not a gold medal or money. The joy of winning and the satisfaction of the effort put forth will be remembered long after the crumpled blue ribbon found years later in a drawer.

For some, however, the prize in winning is so important, that our actions cause us to be vilified, as basketball player LeBron James learned when he packed his bags in Cleveland to move to Miami for an elusive NBA championship ring. If you were living out of the country in 2010 when this happened, his basketball jerseys were burned and the maker of Fathead held a "Benedict Arnold" sale by discounting the $99.99 life-sized images of James to $17.41, the year of Benedict Arnold's birth.

Raising four boys who have participated in a myriad of sports through the years, including soccer, football, basketball, wrestling, baseball, running, skiing and snowboarding, you would think winning should matter a whole lot to me. Indeed, I was raised with a brother who would often repeat the quote, "Winning isn't everything; it's the only thing," **It didn't matter if he was playing basketball, a board game or jacks. If he lost, the game immediately became "best out of three...than best out of five."

Looking back, however, I wonder if there was another reason for winning, because this is the same brother who adores soft serve ice cream and who played for the Dairy Queen baseball team, coached by my father. The spoils of victory for the team after the game included a trip to DQ for free ice cream. My brother had the added bonus of performing for teammates and I still remember him grabbing a logo napkin from the dispenser, turning it over and stating, "Here we have a plain napkin." Then with a swipe behind his backside he would present it, flipped over stating, "I wipe my butt and it's scrumpdillyishus!" So it's possible that the Dairy Queen experience may have been the root cause as to why my brother equated winning with being the only thing, but I think it's just the way he's wired.

Back to the primary reason for the investment of time to allow our boys to participate in sports, and that is for the lessons learned. Topping the list is, of course, the lesson of teamwork. Second on the list is how **not** to act as an adult, whether as a parent (yes I have been there, done that), coach, or referee. Lesson three is the joy of physical activity, the discipline related to it, and the health benefits derived from it. Lesson four happens on a good day, when the planets seem to align, and it is clear that winning travels from being impossible to unlikely, to possible, then probable, and finally achieved!

Scenario: Worst team plays best team, 10-run rule expected in minimum innings. "Wow, we are really fielding well, held them to only two runs in the first inning. We scored three runs? Never thought we'd ever lead this team by a run. Let's enjoy it before the end of the second inning. Good grief, we're still only tied after three innings! We might not get 10-run ruled. We are leading the undefeated team by two runs in the 6th inning? We are cheering our hearts out and their fans are berating their own team, destroying any positive karma the team may have had. All we have to do is hold them and we win- and we do!

Because winning is not in my top three priorities, I have been a mother who regards our "trophy society" as a bit ludicrous. When my twins were in second or third grade, they participated in a basketball tournament, and their team played abysmally. It was Christmas break, so I wasn't keen to sit in a gymnasium for an entire day anyhow, so when their team was eliminated with the obligatory two-loss minimum, you could have shot me out of a rocket and I would not have left the tourney more quickly than I was already leaving. Then the boys showed me their trophies. Their *8th place trophies.*

It truly did not matter to me in any way, shape, or form, that their team placed eighth. It probably should have. My mind was on meals and preparation for company coming for the remainder of the holiday…sled riding, fires in the hearth, hot cocoa with marshmallows and whipped cream, our wedding anniversary, helping my kids pick out my birthday cake, the New Year's Eve menu, not to mention New Year's Day….

Pork, sauerkraut, and mashed potatoes came to a screeching halt in my head as fast as my feet. In front of the poor women manning the tournament table at the front door, I stopped and said, "Oh no. Throw those in this trash. You know that I don't care if you came in 8th place as long as you played your best, but (and I paraphrased the words from the one and only 'Mr. Incredible') we do not celebrate that kind of mediocrity. You will NOT have an 8th place trophy on your shelf." They threw the trophies in the trash to the dismay of the onlookers, and we truthfully by the time we loaded the car, went on our happy way, with highest priority being on the estimated arrival of grandparents, cousins, aunts, and uncles. To this day, one of my sons' favorite teachers, who heard this story later, insists she is going to replace their 8th place trophies that were stripped from their little boy grasps. Since she is like their second mother, and is held in the highest esteem, an 8th place trophy will be permissible from her.

Maybe I am this way because of running. Running is unique. Only one runner wins. The rest of the field can only hope for a personal best if that matters enough to them. So for most runners, simply crossing the finish line at a specified distance is the only prize that matters, which is an understandable one to be sure, and probably the biggest mental hurdle to leap.

And then there is the prize of the experience of the run. This prize has no one cheering on the sidewalks or recording the finish. Lacing up in complete anonymity, stretching, and enjoying mile after mile—for some this is the only true prize.

Without a doubt a runner goes into strict training for a goal. It doesn't take long to realize that a long run after a brownie hot fudge sundae doesn't feel quite the same as one taken following a plate of pasta the night before.

Most races require strict training for many reasons. How you eat, how you sleep, how you hydrate your body and lubricate your thighs matters. Crossing the line for that photo finish documenting the accomplishment with bloodstains on the front of your shirt from not wearing the right frictionless item is rightfully horrifying.

Life is like that. Run in such a way to get the prize. Figuring out what the prize is, now there is a personal journey. What is your prize? Before you go into strict training, you must ask yourself that question. *"What is my prize?"*

Is your prize winning? Making the most money? Having a certain zip code? Driving a certain car? What is your prize in this life? A good exercise is to list the priorities in your life and then see if your living lines up with those priorities. How do you know if your life lines up? Various life coaches say the first two places to look are your calendar and your checkbook. Where does your time and money go? You can see clearly if your training and practice line up with what your prize is.

One of my favorite softball coaches, Ken McDonough, coached me on a team that went to a national tournament in 1980. It is not humility to say my contribution was as the weakest link on the team. Alas, what I lacked in skill, I made up for in desire in playing the game, albeit from right field, and back up at that, and the social aspect of participating with my teammates and being coached by a disciplinarian who made us run. Coach McDonough was perpetually tan, had a smoker's raspy voice, and repeatedly taught us (and I will never forget what he said, only years later learning it was actually a quote from Vince Lombardi – is it a Western Pennsylvania thing or a guy thing to quote Vince Lombardi?) In fact, I'm sure he attributed it to Vince Lombardi, but I heard, "Blah blah blah, blah blah blah great coach, blah blah blah, **Practice does not make perfect. Only perfect practice makes perfect.**"

No matter what I did in life, *I remembered* those words. They went to my very marrow. *Practice does not make perfect. Only perfect practice makes perfect.* When I wanted to be as good as pulmonary technicians at drawing arterial blood gases, those words came back, and when one of the leukemia patients in intensive care requested me to perform the procedure, it was humbling beyond measure.

So what is your elusive prize in the way you live that requires perfect practice-strict training? Let's say having family time is a priority to you, yet when you look at your schedule, you realize you are not spending quality time with your family. An alignment in everyone's schedule needs to occur to accommodate this goal. Perhaps placing a moratorium on Sunday afternoons to have a family dinner and to play games is a way to achieve this goal, but it won't happen without effort.

For many runners, achieving a personal best time or running a marathon is their prize. Running a marathon is a monumental goal for many, and rightfully so because twenty-six and two-tenths miles is *far*. At the age of twenty-four, it was my prize, a seemingly unattainable goal. It wasn't until 1989 when my cousin introduced me to *Jeff Galloway's Book of Running* that I could mentally conceive it for myself, even though I was regularly running ten miles easily and fifty miles in a week.

The mentality in Galloway's book, and his marathon advice, according to my cousin, was that if you can imagine stretching the furthest distance you have run by two miles, and two weeks later doing it again, you can mentally tackle a marathon. My cousin asked a crucial question "So if you run six miles, you can push yourself to complete eight in two weeks, right?" I replied that I could do that. "Fine, then two weeks later, you'll run ten, and so on."

So after scouring the extraordinary book, containing a plethora of running knowledge based upon experience and wisdom, I remember following the training advice for finishing a marathon in under four hours like a recipe and finished the Marine Corps Marathon in 3:59 (this was even before staggered starts were monitored electronically). My brother and his wife rode bicycles around the monuments and cheered me on. They later told me how predictable my appearance became because my pace was steady, which I attribute to the training offered by Galloway. There was no hitting the "wall" because I had already finished a 24-mile run weeks before the race. It was an amazing feeling to finish a goal so desperately prized.

Having bought the book, and twenty more, because they flew off my bookshelf into the hands of others, the same Galloway logic with which my cousin enlightened me was what I shared in 2001 with a woman I met when I ran past her house and her English Mastiff chased me.

Stephanie Daniels went on to become the female champion of the Johnstown, Pennsylvania Marathon in her first marathon and then repeated the feat once again the next and only time she attempted to do so. Years later, Stephanie helped me to attain a prize I didn't realize would be so coveted. It was my slowest time in a 5k race. That's right, my *slowest* time in a 5,000-meter race is probably the only other timed running feat I cherish besides my first marathon.

Together, we worked to organize a group of middle school kids in our district to train and run in the fundraiser organized by our local newspaper, The Daily American. Springtime weather in Pennsylvania can be challenging to say the least, and that year was no exception, so we didn't have the kids quite where we wanted them to be before school let out for the year.

On race day, there were a few of the kids languishing at the halfway mark, one girl in particular. For the remainder of the course, another mom and I stayed with her, spurring her on, and finally finishing just behind her to the cheers of her family. It was glorious. The newspaper printed the times of the race, and there was my name right after the last middle schooler to finish. Bliss.

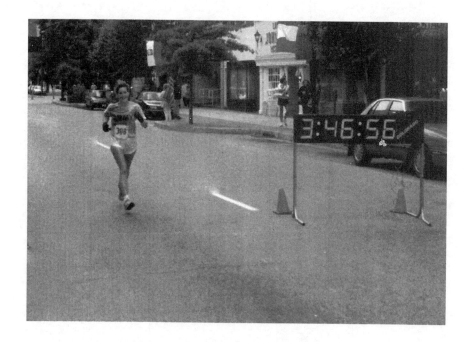

Johnstown YMCA Marathon 1991

A week after the race, someone called to tell me that I was first for my age group, but a mistake had been made in my registration, so I had been classified as a male. They were super apologetic and said they would send my trophy immediately. I told them it was fine I didn't need a trophy, but they sent it anyhow. The trophy I carried in my heart years later was the middle schooler who finished the 5k race!

Pondering for the Road

Determine if you know what your prize is, and if it needs to be reevaluated and revamped; then ask yourself if you are living your life in training or if you need to go into strict training to achieve that prize.

My Prayer for You

My prayer for you is that you open your heart and your mind to what God is calling you heavenward to do, and that you press on towards that goal.

Sustenance for the Road

Therefore I do not run like a man running aimlessly...I myself will not be disqualified for the prize (1 Corinthians 9:26, 27).

How do you want to go forward?

_____

_____

_____

What story do you have to tell about a prize? Share it at whatilearnedwhilerunning.com.

*Perfect Thai Sticky Rice

Soak "sweet rice" in a large pot of water (it will say highly glutenized on the package-available in Asian markets) for at least 12 hours. Drain into a metal colander. Fill the pot 1/3 full with water and place the strainer of rice on top. Bring water to boil. After 10 minutes, stir and sprinkle with salt. Reset timer for 10 minutes. You should need to do this at least one more time. Serve with peanut sauce. I use one can lite coconut milk (not sweetened), one teaspoon red curry paste, ¼ cup brown sugar and ¼ cup peanut butter. Heat and whisk all together.

**For years, I thought Vince Lombardi spoke those words. While reviewing Vince Lombardi quotes, research suggests the person who actually said this was UCLA Bruins football coach Henry Sanders.

6

WAITING

I wait for the LORD, my soul waits,
and in his word I put my hope.
My soul waits for the Lord
more than watchmen wait for the morning,
more than watchmen wait for the morning.
Psalm 130: 5,6

Patience is not the ability to wait,
but the ability to keep a good attitude while waiting.
~Joyce Meyer

One of the most self-disciplined lessons one can learn from running is waiting. Obviously, waiting is counterintuitive to our society's teachings, which seem to feed the entitlement of instant gratification. "Presidents' Day Sale! Zero down, zero financing for 60 months!"

We are impatient in heavy traffic, in grocery lines with more than two people ahead of us, and when our children don't obey what we immediately ask them to do. But all the impatience in the world will not make a lightning storm pass faster so that you may hit the trail after a long day of school or work. Even worse, some storms last for days, and bad winters last for months in Pennsylvania.

However, the art of waiting takes on a whole new level when injured. Normally injuries require waiting that is long enough for healing to take place, but because the specific amount of time is difficult to predict, frustration and stress can result. And when one of the activities utilized to alleviate stress is not feasible, it isn't hard to imagine a cycle of anxiety. Some athletes disregard the healing time and further injure themselves. Most of us are guilty of lacking wisdom at one time or another with regard to allowing an injury the full time to heal. Hopefully, it only takes one time for an injury to worsen, resulting in an even longer waiting time to learn the lesson of patience.

And so you learn to wait, perhaps simply out of necessity or the knowledge that the release will come. Waiting while healing doesn't have to mean doing *nothing,* but it does mean doing nothing regarding the right things. Making constructive use of time by doing other "right things" is an excellent way to pass the time.

Having a reserve of activities for those seasons of waiting is helpful, especially if the injury takes you by surprise. Whether it's a library of books on an e-reader, a basket of yarn for knitting, a stack of Bon Appetit magazines, or a queue of movies, a little imagination might just make you look forward to the interruption of your coveted workout routine.

Even as these words are tweaked in fall 2014, this battle is being waged in my own life. Thanks to a herniated disc, I cannot run. There are a few extra hours in my schedule, which has been overwhelmed recently with football laundry for four boys, not to mention cooking and feeding five boys plus my husband. Add trips to the hospital for my father's open-heart surgery, family commitments, doctors' appointments for my son's fractured arm and another son's dislocated finger and you almost have the picture of my life. Because we live on a farm, taking care of horses, dogs and cats are part of a never-ending list of things to do. It has taken nearly a lifetime to learn this lesson, but even though I would love nothing more than to hit the road, I don't want to miss what God wants me to do with those few precious hours of time.

So I wait. Eventually, if one can learn to accept these disruptions, this patient waiting becomes a way of living, and suddenly standing in a long line of frustrated customers is not so difficult. (Well, unless someone has fifty items in the 8-item or less checkout). Then one day, this transcends to being able to wait for the really important things in life. Waiting for the right job, the right mate, and not getting ahead of God, now there's a challenge. Make no mistake about it; it is a learned response, but it can be done.

It is 1987, and springtime could not come soon enough to Long Island, New York. Running a circuit around Glen Cove, my thoughts are dominated by my decision to soon leave my hospital for a job in the Intensive Care Unit at Long Island Jewish Hospital. It wasn't my preference to leave Glen Cove Community Hospital, but the hospital wanted me to stay on the medical surgical floor through September. Although I enjoyed the interesting mix of the three hallways, one with telemetry patients, one with everything from AIDS patients to diabetics, and the third with post-surgical patients, the critical care unit peaked my interest.

During a recent quiet night for me, and a busy one in the "unit," I was tasked with running units of blood upstairs from the lab. William Casey, the CIA director surrounded with controversy due to the "Iran Contra affair," was hospitalized in the ICU. When I was escalating the steps, two men in dark suits appeared seemingly out of nowhere. Halting my ascent, I showed them what I was delivering, and they were friendly enough and let me pass to enter the excitement of the ICU.

So I was looking forward to that environment in the new hospital and working in the ICU, with the only drawback being that we will be without health insurance for three months, and the overtime work I get to help pay the bills. Jim reassured me that we should be fine; we are young and healthy. Mulling this over as I run along Crescent Beach Road on a favorite route, suddenly a crushing sense of foreboding makes me short of breath. Stopping to bend over and grasp my knees, I reach one arm to my chest trying to determine what in the world is happening to me. The immediate crisis eased, and as I walk a bit, eventually I felt like I could breathe normally. Taking a few steps, the overwhelming realization hits me that I am not meant to take the new job. But I have already turned in my two-week resignation. I manage to trot back home to 15 Titus Road to our second floor apartment we rent from an Italian widow for $800 per month.

Later that day, when Jim returns home from medical school and I prepare for one of my last twelve-hour night shifts, I share the episode from my run as well as my epiphany, and again, he is supportive, but I don't know what to do. "Show me what to do, God," I whisper to myself as I walk into the hospital with nighttime approaching. Shortly after midnight, the most intimidating nursing supervisor is on duty and asks me to come into the break room, the smell of cigarette smoke still pervasive from change of shift report hours earlier. She asks why I'm leaving, and I tell her. She asks if I will stay if I can transfer to our ICU. In a heartbeat I say "yes," knowing without a doubt it's the right decision, without knowing why. The answer was soon revealed.

Fast-forward two months to July 1987. My ears hear what the surgeon is saying, but my brain is not registering. A week before, after an Army Reserve training weekend marred by a dull pain in my abdomen, I drove to meet my husband at the hospital where he was enjoying his first clinical rotation, which happened to be a surgery rotation on a quiet Sunday afternoon.

Suddenly, a sharp pain emanating from my lower back made me lightheaded, and I nearly fainted, so Jim quickly found me a gurney, and after recovering, I drove home to get ready for work. When the bleeding started, I attributed the pain to a severe menstrual cycle, and headed to my shift to discover many interesting patients.

We had a patient with Amyotrophic Lateral Sclerosis (Lou Gehrig's Disease), a patient with Guillian Barre', and that evening, a young man who was septic was my patient. The pain returned as did the lightheadedness, but I was determined to start a 16 gauge IV so that he could quickly receive the necessary intravenous fluids ordered.

The following evening, the pain was so unbearable, my husband brought me to the Emergency Department. It was then that I realized how fortunate we were that we were not without health insurance. The Resident ran tests, took X-Rays, and told us it was a combination of menstrual discomfort and constipation, and that Milk of Magnesia would help. As we were gingerly walking out the door, he called us back, looking very ill at ease. My pregnancy test had come back positive.

An OB/GYN was consulted, and after a painful examination, told us that I was probably in the midst of an actual miscarriage, and that he would order quantified HCG levels, which would probably decline as opposed to doubling every 48 hours during a normal pregnancy.

This indeed occurred, but in addition, over the course of the next five days, my pain increased, as did the lightheadedness to the point of fainting on more than one occasion, all considered "normal" when I called the doctor's office.

When I developed a fever, I was admitted and scheduled for an abdominal ultrasound. Grim-faced, the ultrasound tech apologized at the pressing and prodding as the pain in my bloated abdomen was unrelenting.

Apparently a large mass of undetermined origin was revealed on my ultrasound, so now, one of my favorite surgeons from the ICU was consulted by the OB/GYN to assist in the removal of it. He was reading the surgery consent form and explaining that the actual surgery would depend upon what he actually found, including hysterectomy, colon resection, appendectomy... the list went on.

My husband and I were alone, our families in Pennsylvania. We said our "goodbyes" before I was taken to the Operating Room. Mine was meant to be the last one I might ever say to this man I had married only nineteen months before. I was wheeled away on the gurney. Being put under brought welcome relief from the pain...

I awoke. The first thing I notice is an empty bag of packed red blood cells hanging from my IV pole. The line needs to be flushed with saline, so I reach up, clamp the tubing and open the saline clamp as I had done so many times before for my patients. Never had I done it for myself, though. On the opposite side of my bed, I see my husband in a chair, and as he immediately comes to my bedside and tries to stop me from taking care of the IV. He explains to me that the mass was actually a 2000 cc clot of blood from a ruptured ectopic pregnancy. My fallopian tube did not rupture in the typical way, and I have apparently been bleeding into my abdomen since the pain began. The pain is gone, as is the swelling in my abdomen, which makes sense if the equivalent of a 2-liter bottle of coke was removed. My husband also explains that my hemoglobin and hematocrit were so low that this is my second unit of blood, and I might need more. It doesn't matter. The goodbye wasn't necessary.

"Would people ever divorce if they were forced to say a 'goodbye' to their spouse early in their marriage," I would later ask myself. The goodbye wasn't necessary.

You might think the waiting in this story was getting rid of the pain over those nine days, and you would be right on one level. Right around this time in the eighties, the blood supply in New York was called into question, so it was recommended anyone who had received transfusions undergo testing for the virus that causes AIDS.

Waiting for the results of two tests, six months apart, was waiting on another level. One of the few friends I had in New York, Connie, a fellow nurse from the medical-surgical ward who, along with her husband, Al, was fighting the battle of the disease. So when Al's IV site failed at home on Thanksgiving Day, and she could find no one from the agency to start another so that he could receive his antibiotic, there was no doubt in my mind that I would do it. Helping them helped me during that time, until I was assured the tests were negative. *

But the real waiting came about when it was revealed that if I could not get pregnant, we would have to undergo In-Vitro Fertilization, which at that time had a $10,000 price tag and poor success, in the range of 11%. Some people close to me suggested we sue because of the misdiagnosis for at least the cost of undergoing the procedure a few times. I thought of the check I wrote every year for malpractice insurance on my nursing license, and decided that just because someone can sue doesn't mean they should. Besides, the resident who admitted the reason he didn't consider an ectopic pregnancy was that it didn't seem like I "was in enough pain" certainly learned from his mistake.

Six months after my surgery, with the tender but healing incision from one side of my pelvis to the other, right through my abdominal muscles, my hysterosalpingogram reveals one open fallopian tube, although the functionality of it was unknown. We were to try to get pregnant as soon as possible.

After my Reserve Officer Basic Course in Texas, we headed for Hawaii for three months of medical school rotations for Jim. He wanted exposure at both military and civilian hospitals for internship applications. A national shortage of critical care nurses allowed me to sign with an agency to work at Queen's Medical Center in Honolulu. We spent the hot humid summer working in Pennsylvania, then headed to the relief of mountain air in Colorado through winter, he at Fitzsimons Army Medical Center and I at University Hospital, with a rotation in Pennsylvania for the holidays. We waited. But month after month, the tell tale sign of blood revealed our near future and it didn't include a baby. After one year of "trying" with no success, I was officially infertile.

Being a glass half full person, I tried to look at the bright side. After all, as the primary breadwinner, how would I take time off from work?

My older sister was trying to get pregnant at the same time, and I prayed for that to happen first, anyhow.

The months turned into years. Jim graduated from medical school and we took a belated honeymoon to Ireland, before Jim started his internship. Friends who were married after us were either having children or getting divorced. We waited. My sister finally gave birth to a son, and the relief I felt was overwhelming. Still, acclimating to the insensitive things people would say became a way of life. "Believe me, you don't want children!" or "No wonder you aren't getting pregnant with all the night shifts you both work."

So we went about living, bought a farm, fell in love with four dogs, and traveled. Problems with scar tissue and ovarian cysts prompted another surgery to remove one of my ovaries, and an attempt at microsurgery on the fallopian tubes "since we're in there anyway." The surgeon was so delighted to tell me he gave me a Pfannenstiel or bikini incision, because the first incision cut through my abdominal muscles. "Great, now I have two scars," I thought but thanks to God, vanity went out the window long ago, because I will never have a flat abdomen. Still, I had peace over the whole thing, a sort of hope.

In the King James Version, Isaiah 40:31 says, But they that wait upon the LORD shall renew their strength; they shall mount up with wings as eagles; they shall run, and not be weary; and they shall walk, and not faint. The New International Version translation uses the word "hope" for wait. But those who hope in the LORD will renew their strength. They will soar on wings like eagles; they will run and not grow weary, they will walk and not be faint. Learning to wait is a lot like not giving up hope.

We went on living. I ran my first marathon, worked in an Emergency Department, back to Intensive Care, and then had a foray into management and home care. Jim finished his five-year surgical residency, applied for Vascular Surgery fellowships and we both landed at The Cleveland Clinic Foundation. On our tenth wedding anniversary, we sat with Dr. Jeffrey Goldberg as he outlined what we believed we already knew. We would have to undergo in-vitro.

A whole book could be written about the waiting with infertility. To understand the anguish, you can visit a true story thousands of years old. Read about the strife and heartache of Hannah in First Samuel. Add the surrender of dignity and modesty to numerous gynecological procedures, blood tests, intramuscular injections, and ultrasounds, and you have a glimpse of the roller coaster ride. Plummeting into the abyss occurs every time you see blood revealing once again that you are not expecting.

Appointment after appointment was made, ultrasounds performed, blood tests were taken, $2000 worth of medications were ordered, and I was ready to start the process. Running helped me to keep my mind clear and stress at bay. When the IVF nurses called and left a message on our apartment phone answering machine that we would have to postpone another cycle because the embryologist would be away, I completely and utterly lost it. Standing in my kitchen on Latimore Street, I was hysterically crying so loudly that I'm sure the tenants on the second and third floor heard me. Eleven years of emotion finally had their release. Finally, after the flood subsided, and my husband spoke reason to me that we had waited this long we could wait a little longer, I surrender. I call the nurse the next day to learn the new date, and she flippantly says, "Oh never mind, I thought you were one of our ICSI (intra-cytoplasmic sperm injection-a special procedure) patients." All of that sorrow was not for nothing; it needed to be purged.

The surrender mindset also was necessary as the lack of control over the process took over. Intramuscular injections were required nightly, and my husband, as a physician, was not particularly adept at giving them. Yes, ouch. However, one night, he called to say he wouldn't be home in time and it was too late to arrange for one of my nurse friends to administer. I would have to stick the 1½-inch needle in my own thigh. It took me a while to work up the courage, but inspired by a news report of a man in Pennsylvania who recently amputated a limb to free himself from under a tree, I did it.

Surrender was also essential because my doctor was never the one who seemed to be on duty when it was time to have my intravaginal ultrasounds. It was a young female physician who reminded me of Carrie Fisher from Star Wars with a light saber the first time I saw her-not particularly warm and fuzzy. (I later grew to adore this woman). Check your dignity and control at the patient desk, please.

The last concern was that Jim was sitting for his Oral Surgery Boards on September 11th, the second most important exam in his life thus far to become Board Certified in General Surgery. This was the only day that would be inconvenient to undergo the procedure, but at least the exam was offered in Cleveland as opposed to Chicago. Naturally, this happened to be the day we were scheduled as the ideal day according to all my levels and measurements. The egg retrieval was a success, and ten embryos were available. Two days later three of them were transferred and the rest were frozen. We waited again.

Two weeks later, I had a positive pregnancy test, but would have to wait another few weeks for an ultrasound. Ten days days before that was scheduled, I was standing in the pet store with my yellow lab and felt the familiar rush of blood. I made it home and crumpled to the floor in grief. The nurse on the phone advised me to stop in the department on my way to work the next morning. There on the screen was a tiny beating heartbeat in our baby's little body. I made my Hannah offering then and there. Our child would be God's. In 1997, Paul was born.

It would have been so easy to turn him into a god, but we simply couldn't. He was a treasure we waited a long time to hold. In his book, *The Pursuit of God*, A.W. Tozer says, "*We are often hindered from giving up our treasures to the Lord out of fear for their safety. This is especially true when those treasures are loved relatives and friends. But we need have no such fears. Our Lord came not to destroy but to save. Everything is safe which we commit to Him, and nothing is really safe which is not committed.*"

Just because you wait for a treasure for a long time, doesn't mean you have the right to turn it into a god. Whether it's a new home, the love of your life, or the education you dreamed about, the question to ask yourself is if these things are God's or gods.

Two years later, our twins were born, and when they did something outrageous, my husband and I would look at one another and quip, "freezer burn." One of my favorite verses, Psalm 37:4, says, "*Delight yourself in the LORD and He will give you the desires of your heart.*" I didn't deserve to have any more desires, because of the delight that ranneth over, but I did, which was to not leave any embryos behind. Two more transfers of two resulted in pregnancies, but both sets of twins were miscarried. Still, the peace to have given them a chance at life was profound beyond words. Then the unexplainable happened. Fifteen years since the ruptured ectopic, we had a pregnancy "on our own" (a boy with heart defects and Downs' syndrome whose heart stopped beating in utero). When the inexplicable occurred again at the age of 38, my physician said, "You are the most fertile infertile patient I have ever known." Still there was much waiting because we were to anticipate the same devastating outcome as the other spontaneous pregnancy, but it never happened. A healthy baby boy survived who brings us much joy daily.

However, the irony is not lost on me that the very children for whom my husband and I waited so many years are often the very people with whom I become most exasperated in waiting...for them to pick up wet towels, put glasses in the dishwasher, or take out the trash.

Even now when reading stories about couples' infertility and the pain and heartache they endure for a few months or years, it is even more convicting to attribute the joy, patience and trust during my nearly twelve years of waiting to the waiting that running taught me and is teaching me to this day.

Pondering for the Road

Ask yourself exactly what you are waiting for and consider that there is something to be learned in this season of waiting, and if you have been using time efficiently while you wait....Wait for the LORD; be strong and take heart and wait for the LORD. Psalm 27:14

My Prayer for You

I pray that you will wait upon the Lord, and hope in the Lord. I pray that your strength would be renewed, if only for today...and that in His Word, you put your hope, more than watchmen wait for the morning.

Sustenance for the Road

I waited patiently for the LORD; he turned to me and heard my cry. Psalm 40:1

How do you want to go forward?

_____

_____

_____

Do you have a story to tell about waiting?
Tell it at whatilearnedwhilerunning.com

*Al and Connie lost their battle with AIDS.

7

REST

"Come to me all you who are weary and burdened
and I will give you rest."
Matthew 11:28

And he saw that rest was good.
Genesis 49:15 KJV

It is with deliberate intention that this chapter on rest follows the chapter on waiting. Rest is different from waiting, although try telling that to a young mother yearning for her baby to go down for his nap. When my twins were babies, and there seemed to be a perpetual cup of coffee reheated in the microwave (yuck!), I used to always say I was so tired my hair hurt.

We all know rest is devalued in our culture. From teenagers to executives, we seem to measure our worth by how much we go go go. Once I was so pressed for time that I went straight to the beauty salon after running (without showering) so that I could utilize the miniscule time to get my desperately overgrown eyebrows waxed and my bangs (overgrown to cover my bushy eyebrows) cut. (As an aside, when your sons borrow your tweezers, it should trigger the same mommy radar that goes off when they simultaneously look in the dining room corner when you ask, "So what happened to the toad you had yesterday?") So I rushed in and the sweet Japanese beautician welcomed me and took me to the waxing station, and I explained my relief that I had just enough time to accomplish getting both things done. After she finished my eyebrows, applying the most soothing salve, she said in broken English, "You want me do you moustache, too?" My eyes flew open and I could only stammer, "Uh... yes you'd better." There was no time to have my bangs cut but my conclusion was that when someone defines you as having a moustache, that's what you get for rushing around in frenzy.

When our friends from Argentina were flying home with small children, an issue with the airplane forced the pilots to divert the plane to a small airport. When the plane was airborne ready, the passengers and crew were forced to wait until the staff awoke from their afternoon nap. As you can imagine, when they told this story to people from the United States, the response was incredulity. That is an incomprehensible scenario in the United States. Think Chicago O'Hare.

Athletes who disregard rest in their regimen usually find themselves regretting this practice as much as those who undertrain. Because the activity is so beneficial, it is easy to continue to run day after day, without adequate recovery, but then legs feel as though they can barely be lifted and sluggishness prevails. Weariness can demand rest from exercise as muscle fibers beg for restoration. We could take a lesson from preschool classes by scheduling rest.

Scheduling days of rest from running is essential to continuing to enjoy the regimen. When I was young, it seemed to be convenient and optimal to run five days a week with two days of rest. I have no proof that it helped to prevent injuries, but I've had few ailments related to running in nearly thirty-five years. Now that my joints and muscles are reaching the half-century mark, I have found that even more days of rest are essential, so my practice is to reverse the regimen, running two or three long runs and resting the other days.

The apostle, John, tells one of the most multi-layered stories in Scripture, when Jesus talks to a woman at the well, as he is traveling from Judea to Galilee via Samaria. Included in the passage is that Jesus was weary from his journey and *rested*.

Jesus, tired as he was from the journey, sat down by the well. John 4:6

So even if you don't believe Jesus is the Son of God, you have to admit he is one of the most significant figures in all history, but were you aware that he needed rest? And if one of the singularly dominant prominent influences in the history of the world were not indefatigable, why would we think we are?

In addition to rest, in terms of importance, is recreation. We seem to forget they go hand in hand, and our lives suffer when we lack both. The military knew it was important and used to call the breaks R&R (rest and recreation). Americans work themselves silly (been there, done that), collapse into bed, and then have stress-induced insomnia, leading to an exhausted society. Then we rush to the nearest Starbucks (not being critical – I love Starbucks!) to get the caffeine we need to get through the day. But still, we are tired.

If it doesn't seem to be a concern, one needs to look at some of the most devastating events caused by human error with the influence of sleep deprivation, including the Three Mile Island nuclear reactor meltdown, as well as the groundings of both the Exxon Valdez cruise ship and the Star Princess.

When you exercise, you especially need rest. This lesson was learned quite embarrassingly when I was in high school, and asked to babysit for the Fontanesi family the evening after a track invitational. Although I had initially declined because I knew I would be tired, the parents were in a bind and said it would be just for a few hours and that they wouldn't be late.

So after being outside all day in the cold and wind, the two little girls undoubtedly were not impressed with my lack of energy in terms of being "fun." Even with snacks, the fatigue was descending upon me. After the girls' bedtime, I found myself splashing water on my face, pacing, then did what every high schooler did at 11:30 pm and turned on Saturday Night Live. Eddie Murphy was my favorite cast member, although I normally fell asleep during the commercials before the musical guest (if I was with my friends, I was the one who got their hand stuck in a bowl of warm water), so I was hoping the Fontanesis would be home soon.

When they weren't home by midnight, I knew I was in trouble. At some point, I sat on the couch and was OUT. They were home shortly thereafter and did not have a house key, so they knocked and rang the doorbell, but I was in such a deep sleep, that I did not awaken. At first they were afraid to be too noisy and frighten the girls, but eventually were banging on the window nearest to where they could see me sound asleep, to no avail. Next, they drove to a local convenience store to call the house phone, and still I slept through the ringing.

Subsequently, and this has become legendary lore in the realm of local babysitting stories, Mr. Fontanesi hoisted his petite wife onto the porch roof so that she could crawl through an unlocked window. Just as she started to descend the stairs, my highly perceptive, super acute babysitting sonar went off and I leapt off the couch and shouted the obvious, "I fell asleep!" As Mrs. Fontanesi unlocked the door, they were both very gracious about it, and actually teased about how much fun they had in the roof caper.

I never took a babysitting job after an invitational again let alone a track meet. And when I entered the world of sleep deprivation from working twelve-hour nights, it taught me how quickly one can succumb to falling asleep when one shouldn't.

A 2010 article from U.S. News and World Report suggests that driving while sleepy is equivalent to driving drunk. The Centers for Disease Control concurs, listing less attentive drivers, slower reaction times and decision-making ability according to a 2012 study in the journal of Accident Analysis and Prevention. The National Highway Traffic Safety Administration estimates drowsy driving causes 2.5% of fatalities in crashes.

My mother raised six kids, and contributed to the upbringing of countless others, so in the chaos of laundry and cooking, dirty dishes and driving kids to activities, she had a few gems for rest and recreation. For rest, nearly every day she would turn on the Days of Our Lives soap opera. She would be asleep by the time the first hourglass appeared and the music played. Her power nap lasted until the second hourglass appeared and we were told to stay tuned to the second half of Days of Our Lives. Often my mother would jump up to attend to some chore such as taking laundry off the clothesline. Undoubtedly, she never actually watched a full episode of her "favorite" daytime show.

For recreation, my mother participated in a variety of endeavors, from taking cake-decorating classes and ceramics classes to playing cards. Many Friday and Saturday nights found my parents and other couples or just us kids around the table playing spades or pinochle. Additionally, since my father was involved in a plethora of athletic pursuits, including coaching and tennis, my mother found a walking partner and the two of them could be found many late afternoons walking around the school district grounds and through town. I was in college when I learned her dear friend had died, along with her mother in a wintry crash as they were driving home from the hair salon. My mother never had another walking partner.

Now my mother walks alone, and still continues to this day. Using Nordic walking sticks, highly popular in Europe, she travels throughout the streets of our hometown. Additionally she utilizes the sunglasses she was given after her cataract surgery. One day she was lamenting to my sister and me that she just couldn't believe no one stopped her to inquire about her walking sticks, going on and on about how people are just not curious but should know how wonderful they are. My sister pulled me into the kitchen and said, "I'm pretty sure no one stops her because they think she's blind." For a second the image had to register in my mind of my mother storming through town with those walking sticks and wrap-around dark lenses and what folks must think as they try to figure out how she can go so fast, and I could tell my sister was waiting for the fully emerged image as we both erupted into hysterical laughter.

So it was extremely beneficial to witness how restorative rest and recreation was for my mother. She wouldn't be labeled a happy person, but she was as happy as she could be, with those intentional activities.

She really hit the jackpot with the addition of knitting and crocheting, because she can sit and relax, and watch old movies as her creativity is allowed to flow. I am quite sure she has given away a thousand afghan blankets through the years. No one who knows Elaine Stewart is freezing in western Pennsylvania!

So in terms of recreation, Robert Schuller said, "What would you attempt to do if you knew you could not fail?" What would you do? Would you learn to kayak? Take up knitting? One of my friends began painting and became outstanding at Hawaiian landscapes. On the other hand, despite numerous classes my own painting skills are pitiful. But I don't have to wonder....

So back to rest. Since we are so great at making schedules, one solution to getting rest is to put it on the calendar. There is a movement in our country called Sabbath-keeping, which many people find to be extremely rewarding. Much like the Sundays of yesteryear, the day is preserved and set aside as a day of rest. If it is on a Sunday, attending worship, having dinner with family or friends, relaxing, and taking a walk are all aspects of this. Avoiding activities requiring others to work is also a component for some, although I seem to be guilty of needing to pick up just one more thing from the grocery store on those days. Many pastors and priests, who after all work on Sundays, take their day of rest Monday or another day during the week.

The danger, as in all good things, is to become legalistic. Years ago on a Sunday afternoon, during a particularly stressful time, the most restorative and rejuvenating thing I could do was to take a long glorious afternoon run, which would have fulfilled the purpose to restore me when one of my neighbors drove up alongside me and shouted, "Don't you know it's the Sabbath? You shouldn't be doing that." He was not joking. On the flip side, upon apologizing once to a grocery clerk for being yet another customer in line, she bathed me in grace when she said, "Don't be sorry! If I didn't have these hours I couldn't pay all my bills!"

Having been a registered nurse who worked twelve-hour shifts on Sundays for many years, and with a husband who is a surgeon who must see and operate on patients on Sundays, not to mention at least one son with youth sports from time to time on Sundays, we treasure and appreciate those times of rest and preserve them when we can. Sometimes we have to wait for a good snowstorm to receive the blessing of true rest, and oh, is it savored.

Some people take a rest day a different day of the week. Why is it important? Is it just to benefit us physically? I don't believe so. There is a benefit that all the clamor of our lives prevents us from experiencing and it is written in Psalm 46:10. *"Be still and know that I am God."* It's so reassuring that it doesn't say, "Put your nose to the grindstone and know that I am God," or, "Spin your wheels and run frantically around and know that I am God." If we want to know God, we need to be still.

One of the most profound questions I have ever heard asked was by Rick Warren, author of *The Purpose Driven Life,* in a study that accompanied the book *The Relationship Principles of Jesus,* by Tom Holladay. The study, named *40 Days of LOVE,* contains sessions you would expect in a study about love, such as "Love is Patient, Love is Kind." However, one particular session struck a nerve with me and that was "The Habits of a Loving Heart." I was expecting the takeaway points to be something like helping a neighbor in need, etc. The number one point in "The Habits of a Loving Heart" was *Develop habits that refresh me physically.* And number one under that point was *rest*.

In the video session, and I am paraphrasing, but Warren essentially asks how important is rest to God? Well, important enough to put it in the Ten Commandments along with not committing adultery. And indeed, Exodus 20:9,10 say *Six days you shall labor and do all your work, but on the seventh day is a Sabbath to the LORD your God. On it you shall not do any work.*

In case you were wondering, the second point Warren makes in "The Habits of a Loving Heart" is *Develop habits that recharge me emotionally.* These include *solitude, recreation and laughter.* One of the funny quotes he states in the video is, *"Some of you have so many irons in the fire that you're putting out the fire!"*

So learning the lesson of the importance of rest and recreation is crucial. You don't need to take a mental inventory to ask yourself what you do for rest and recreation and how often you do it, to know that you aren't doing it enough. Put it on the schedule!

Pondering for the Road

When was the last time you felt truly and genuinely rested? When was the last time you practiced the art of doing nothing?

My Prayer for You

My prayer for you is that you will find the rest you so desperately need, whether a 20 minute catnap daily or to the very marrow of your soul.

Sustenance for the Road

but those who hope in the LORD will renew their strength. They will soar on wings like eagles; they will run and not grow weary, they will walk and not be faint. Isaiah 40:31

How do you want to go forward?

_____

_____

_____

Share your story regarding rest at whatilearnedwhilerunning.com.

8

Forgiveness

I don't always know when I'm right, but I sure know
when I'm wrong. These are critical times...
~1981 song *Critical Times* by Quarter Flash

Forgetting what is behind and straining toward what
is ahead, I press on toward the goal to win the prize
for which God has called me heavenward...
Philippians 3:13,14

What could one learn from God about forgiveness while running? Think about the last time you did or said something that made you later think, "stupid, stupid, stupid." Or has someone ever told you that you said or did something that had been offensive when you had no idea that you had done so and furthermore, that what you did was completely unintentional?

If you are excluded from any of these scenarios, all I can say is that it must be great to be you! Skip to the next chapter. As for me, when it comes to what I have done and what I have failed to do, as I tell my children, "I made mistakes yesterday, will undoubtedly make mistakes today, and don't plan to make them tomorrow, but more than likely will." Though still a work in progress, through running, an understanding of heaps of forgiveness bestowed upon me has resulted in my own heart forgiving more readily.

It's a gloriously sunny summer day, so when I reach the shady mile stretch of my run in sunglasses, there are few patches of sunlight streaming down through the thick canopy of green foliage. Since my bladder isn't what it used to be, and there are no cars on this stretch of road, I duck into the forest for a quick pit-stop. Resuming my pace, as I hear cars approaching, I suddenly hear a loud voice over a walkie-talkie announcing, "There are four cars, and the last one is a blue Ford pick-up." I must have jumped two feet in the air from being so startled!

Having never seen the road crew sign operator, suddenly the bright orange and yellow vest was very noticeable, and I realize that this person certainly saw me as I approached, then disappeared into the woods, and emerged adjusting my shorts! What I should have felt was overly embarrassed, I couldn't help but laugh hysterically at the scene that poor person just witnessed, and chuckled the whole way home.

When I was younger, that situation would have replayed over and over in my mind with humiliation afresh. No doubt it's difficult to forget things we do that are just plain stupid, or offensive, or wrong. Or things others have done to us.

During large races, the ubiquitous "runners' tissue" (when the best way to clear a nostril is to press on the other side of your nose and blow hard) is something that inadvertently, yet offensively can strike even as you plod along innocently. "Sorry!" is a word readily heard during race events. But not everyone who hurts you is sorry.

In 1985, while jogging in place at an intersection in Lebanon, Pennsylvania, waiting for the light to turn, a car of teenagers drove so closely that one of the boys slapped me on my rear end. Aside from the pain, the shock was astonishing. In the aftermath of hearing laughter, processing the offense took a few miles. Years later when my godchild, Jessica White, started running, she wrote a poem entitled, *Running With Rednecks* that reminded me of that day, and also told me that she, too had endured offenses from time to time on the road. In my case, just because an apology wasn't extended, forgiveness was possible, so moving forward was the best direction to choose.

Sometimes we choose the wrong direction all on our own. It was 1986 when my husband and I were running in a wooded area in New Jersey and nature called (again ducking into the woods), and not having the poison ivy identification background that was necessary at the time, the mistake was one that stayed with me for two itchy weeks. The bonus lesson that was learned is that no one wakes up saying "Thank God I don't have poison ivy." But once you do have even one bout of poison ivy, it is a thanksgiving that is not hard to profess.

Another situation in which runners find themselves taking life for granted is when dogs are encountered during an outing.

It took me thirty years to be significantly bitten by a dog. Thanks to a love of dogs, usually just stopping and talking with my hand outstretched and palm up has been enough to manage a canine friend in chase. In 1986, my brother-in-law, Davey, fresh out of 82nd Airborne training taught me a useful tactic when we were pursued and nearly attacked by a viciously snarling German Shepherd dog. I cowered behind my husband as Davey whipped around and stomped his foot pointing at the dog and shouted "NO!" It was enough to startle the dog and he took a step back. Davey took another step and repeated his gesture. The dog continued to hesitantly back his way home, still barking, but no longer even attempting to follow us. When I was in awe of how he handled the situation and that we escaped a seemingly inescapable situation, he explained that every dog knows the word, "no." Still, it was a delivery technique that was a useful tool on the road.

So back to the day when two dogs gave chase while passing the neighbor's house. After making friends and petting a dog that our neighbor was watching, I turned to continue on my run after thinking sufficient attention was given, and boy was it startling and surprising to realize that the dog bit me on the butt! He even drew blood!

What I am trying to convey is that someone or something has hurt every adult person on the planet, and as long as we're in these human bodies, you can be darn sure each of us has hurt someone as well. Moreover, who can say they have not made a mistake that was personally detrimental? So much in life can haunt us to dwell and replay over and over in our minds these experiences.

Because we "remember" so clearly, just as these incidents are recalled, the way to forget what is behind is to strain to what is ahead.

Running has a way of helping to forget what is behind, but our "behinds" can be so big (you're thinking, *speak for yourself, right?*), especially when they are slapped, bitten, or covered in poison ivy.

So what is your "behind"? What would you wish to have in a place of forgiveness and peace so that you can approach what is ahead with a fresh approach? Is it a financial hardship, maybe even bankruptcy? Or a divorce that still haunts you? The list is endless: an adulterous affair, addiction, job termination, abortion, physical and emotional abuse, bullying, eating disorder, depression, cutting, death of a loved one, etc. Each of these require legitimate time in order to cope, but should not keep us captive to our graves.

The situations we find hardest to forgive tell us a lot about ourselves. Some people hold a grudge forever if someone else inadvertently does something without even realizing that it was an offense. We have to accept that even if people don't forgive us, God does.

Some people think when someone hurts you financially, it's unforgivable. When an unscrupulous contractor put us in a terrible financial situation after installing an entire expensive geothermal system that didn't work (the bedrooms were 53 degrees in winter with heat on and 90 degrees in summer with air-conditioning, and our "energy-efficient" electric bills were $1000/ month). The system had to be replaced and reconfigured, including the entire ductwork and air handlers, not to mention all the copper pipes and other plumbing issues. Do you want to know how much it costs to replace an expensive system correctly? Twice as much as the original system. Our closest friend from college (who manages wealth) blanched when I said, "Well it's only money." We could have sued, but didn't, and the person who finally figured out how to fix the system said he wouldn't have fixed it if we had filed a lawsuit, so it was a good thing. Besides, the next homeowner that wound up in the same situation with the unscrupulous contractor did get lawyers involved, and yet he burned with anger and unforgiveness and ended up very sick. And despite our hardship, God continued to provide enough that we were able to give more than we had ever given of our time, talents and treasure. Our pain was in the proper perspective.

So much pain can result in even more pain, unless we strain toward what is ahead.

In *My Utmost For His Highest,* Oswald Chambers explains it best, *"Our yesterdays present irreparable things to us; it is true that we have lost opportunities which will never return, but God can transform this destructive anxiety into a constructive thoughtfulness for the future. Let the past sleep, but let it sleep on the bosom of Christ."*

In his epistle to the Philippians, Paul writes that he strains toward the goal to win the prize for which God has called him heavenward. He writes that he hasn't taken hold of it. He doesn't say he just rushes forward and attains it, but that he *strains* toward it, admitting full well he doesn't have all the answers, but he still presses on.

When the Boston Marathon bombing occurred, the scenario seemed unimaginable. It was yet another moment in time that recently emerged where everyone remembers exactly where they were and what they were doing when they heard the news. My sons and I were walking around the Coal Miner's Café in Jennerstown, Pennsylvania to volunteer at the annual fundraiser to benefit the Somerset County Blind Center, when we received a text from my nephew, a student at Dickinson College.

My *first thought* was that it couldn't possibly be runners who did this. I *needed* to know it wasn't. As I walked into the door, the owner, Betty Rhoads, was on the phone with a reporter who was familiar with our community because of 9/11 and the Quecreek mine rescue. He wanted to speak to people in the community about their reaction to the news, so Betty handed me the phone. I tried to explain to him that I didn't know anything except what I had learned from my nephew. The reporter told me he was trying to gauge reaction from across the nation and wanted to know if I felt like, as a Somerset County 9/11 resident, "Here we go again." I could only answer as someone who had run marathons, never conceiving the finish line to be a dangerous place to be, beyond finishing the 26.2 miles (although I was thinking about photographers who have captured runners collapsing and losing control of their bowels, but didn't say that), and no one was more surprised than I when my quotes appeared in the USA Today and in a special electronic edition that Time did about that horrible day.

So many heroes emerged from that day, and continue to press on, despite the seemingly justifiable place of remaining in a state of unforgiveness. Even though the city of Boston had to heal and the nation had to heal from the heinous act, the pain and suffering endured by the families who lost loved ones, and by those who lost limbs to the bombings is almost unbearable to perceive.

How do you forgive someone who molests your precious niece? How do your neighbors go on when a drunk driver has killed their child? I don't have the answers for such evil. In fact, I have to confess that in 1989 when I worked in a Medical Intensive Care Unit in Denver, Colorado, the staff held a "deep-fried" potluck picnic at work the night Ted Bundy was electrocuted, and without any hesitation I brought fried bananas and ice cream. In college, one of the true frightening stories retold to me was of the murders Bundy carried out against Chi Omega college students in Florida. Then reading about how Bundy lured young women posing as an injured man needing to be rescued (for some reason I had thought they were joggers but have since seen no proof to support that assumption), but my "judgment" was complete. *

So I don't have the answers for such evil, and do know sometimes life is just so heartbreaking that it's hard to go forward. When a niece you are trying to protect in the sanctuary of your home gets stripped out of your arms to return to a toxic environment, sometimes all we can do is to stand or fall to our knees. Still, God can call us heavenward in ways we never imagined.

On Sunday, September 9, 2001, while taking a family walk on our farm with our twins in backpack carriers, we noticed one tree in full fall foliage regalia amongst a hundred acres of green trees. It was so beautiful we took photos of it. I promised my 4-year old that we would hike back two days later to pick some of the leaves and iron them into placemats for the friends he left behind in Hawaii to show them what Autumn looked like. We had the Radio Flyer wagon ready to go when my husband called for me to turn on the television, telling me an airplane had earlier hit one of the World Trade Center buildings, and then a second one hit the other. When my son started asking questions about what happened to the buildings on fire, I knew I had to get him away from the television and we headed around the house to the front yard. We watched as the largest airplane we had ever seen pass over our farm at such a low altitude went over our heads. It was so low we could make out windows.

*Earlier that summer my son and I saw a very small airplane circle over our farm and we thought it was strange the pilot didn't wave or have a camera like most small aircraft we see. Turns out, the pilot had made an emergency crash-landing nearby after flying over our farm. A photo of the crash made the front page of the local newspaper with an article about his emergency landing. So, on what we now call 9/11, my son asked me if we were going to see **this** plane on the newspaper like the other one.*

I was shaking, filled with trepidation, and told my son I didn't know but that maybe the plane was going to land on Route 219 or at the Johnstown airport, praying to myself that the runway was long enough. I told him that we needed to pray for those people on the plane that they would be safe and would get home to their families, and that God would be with them. For an instant

I was reminded of the feeling I had in 1986, after a cold January run at Penn State with my friend Meg McGroarty, when we walked into her apartment to see the replay of the Space Shuttle Challenger explosion. One of my husband's roommates, Steve, from 101 Norle Ranch, in Lemont, Pennsylvania, had applied for the teacher position that was ultimately won by Christa MacAuliffe. Life was brought back to reality by my twins tumbling over each other to get into the wagon, so we went to the tree. On return, I quietly tried to look at the television, and learned that a flight had gone down in Somerset County, and I watched as the second tower collapsed.

The phone lines were already starting to jam when my husband called from the hospital, I told him we had seen the plane before it went down, although I could tell he didn't believe the news. He advised me to get milk and bread at the local dairy, Rolling Acres, and when I told the owner that we think we saw the plane, he told me, "I bet you did, because one of my customers ran back in from the parking lot saying a plane just flew over, and it wasn't long after the news said a plane went down out by Indian Lake." Before long we learned it was United Flight #93, down in a field near Shanksville.

Was there a day better described by Ephesians 6:12 as stated, "For our struggle is not against flesh and blood, but against rulers, against the authorities, against the powers of this dark world and against the spiritual forces of evil in the heavenly realms." We are told in the previous verse to put on the full armor of God so that we can take our stand against the devil's schemes. Four more times in the chapter it says to stand. 9/11 was a day where that was the best we could do: to take our stand, to stand our ground, to stand, to stand firm. We are not advised to enter into a footrace with the devil, just told to simply stand. Take a stand. The heroes of Flight 93 took a stand.

As with most United States citizens, that day is forever etched in my memory, but for years I grieved over the memory of standing in my front yard with my little boys, unable to do anything but pray. It wasn't until the tenth anniversary of the attacks as I was replaying that day in my mind during a run that God blessed me with a new insight, perhaps because prayer is more and more important to me as the years go by. What I realized was that we were some of the last people on this planet to *pray* for those on Flight 93. We prayed them to the hereafter. It wasn't eloquent and it certainly wasn't pretty as I bent down on shaky knees and fought tears to not scare my oldest son while two blonde toddlers battled over the wagon.

All we could do was to stand and we did pray and that's not nothing. It's *something.* Oswald Chambers' words regarding prayer are many, but my favorite are these from October 17th of *My Utmost, "Prayer does not fit us for the greater works; prayer* is *the greater work."*

We don't always get it right, and even when we do get it right, we can still beat ourselves up. But there is a purpose for our lives and we need to strain toward what is ahead, rather than dwelling in the past of whatever we dragged our sorry butts into or what was done to them. Consider what you may be called to do, and if you are dwelling in a past patch of poison ivy into which you plopped yourself, concerned about critics and what they will say about you, I can only encourage you with what I call the "Fort McHenry principle."

During a trip to lovely Inner Harbor, Baltimore, Maryland, we visited Fort McHenry and the site where the very flag flew during the Battle of Baltimore in the War of 1812, that inspired Francis Scott Key from his vantage point aboard the British ship, the HMS Tonnant. After Key penned the "Defence of Fort M'Henry," it was published in a local newspaper, eventually accompanied by music and the rest is quite literally history. The Star Spangled Banner still brings me to tears no matter where I hear it. However, one of the most interesting facets of the historical site to me was that Key was widely criticized after his initial fame or whatever is the equivalent in 1814.

There were people who were criticizing Key, stating that with the smoke and darkness, and from the proximity of the ship's position in the harbor, he could not have seen the flag still flying the next morning, signifying that Fort McHenry had survived the British onslaught. If social media had been alive and well in those days, the attack Key would have endured would have been worse than the battle itself, I'm certain. So here are my takeaways as I mused and jogged around the Inner Harbor:

1. There will *always* be critics no matter what good thing you do, and just in case you write words that will be as profound as our national anthem, disregard what these people say about you.
2. If you are like me, there is nothing worse that people can think or say about you than you have thought or said about yourself. So tell them to get in the back of the line, you were there first in terms of critic emeritus, and forward, ho.

3. People in Baltimore (or at least around the Inner Harbor) are *really, really nice people.* Seriously, when you are a Pittsburgh Steelers fan, you just don't realize that! Ok, that doesn't have to do with Fort McHenry, but it's still a profound takeaway.

Forgiveness of self and others can be an elusive but attainable achievement. Many variations exist of the common but powerful quote, *"Unforgiveness is like drinking poison and hoping the other person gets sick."* Personally I think it's like fishing. You cast your line, flinging it far, far, away in a blaze of sunshine and reflecting waters. Then after a long while you slowly start reeling it back in, with nothing but emptiness. The day comes when you know you have cut the line once and for all when you feel in your heart you are not going to reel it again.

In the 18th chapter of the gospel of Matthew, Peter, asks Jesus how many times he should forgive his brother, because in that day rabbis taught that you should forgive, but only three times. It's one more generous than the mentality that if you offend me once, shame on you, but if you offend me twice, shame on me. So the lesson of the day was that after three strikes, you're out. So Peter, demonstrating how astonishingly comprehending he is of Jesus' teaching regarding forgiveness queries, "Up to seven times?"

In my opinion, Jesus' reply may be as important to the foundation of who Peter becomes after his three denials before the crucifixion. In the New International Version, Jesus says, "I tell you, not seven times, but seventy-seven times." Jesus' reply in the King James Version is, "Until seventy times seven." I have heard some who do the multiplication in that translation; regardless, whether you believe Christ is saying 77 or 490, He is telling Peter in my estimation, "You're not even close, fisherman. You have to cut the line clean over and over and over." If Peter didn't get it then, there is no doubt in my mind he got it when, as Luke writes in his gospel immediately after the rooster crowed, *The Lord turned and looked straight at Peter. 22:61*

The thought of getting that look makes me cringe for Peter's sake, even thousands of years after the fact. Certainly, recounting that earlier lesson with Jesus had to help him to not only to accept God's forgiveness, but the more difficult task of forgiving himself. So all of that to say, that if it's difficult for the man who became the foundation for establishing

Christ's church on Earth after His resurrection, of course it is going to be a struggle for us. Thankfully, the gift of mercy extended to us, as to Peter, teaches us to be merciful.

My dear friend, Susan Moore, used to say to her triplet girls when she taught them to say they were sorry for something one had done to another, "Now you have the hard part. You have to forgive her." Not easy, but possible, and thanks be to God, the Father, Son and Holy Spirit are there to help us.

Years earlier her husband, Richard Moore, wrote me a poem from Champaign, Illinois, while in a Colorectal Surgery Fellowship, to help me with grieving for my friend, Connie (mentioned in Chapter 6) and forgiving myself for not making her a quilt for the AIDS quilt project before she died, something I had longed to do. I call it *Connie's Quilt,* although he sent it to me untitled on the envelope.

Connie's Quilt, by Richard A. Moore, MD, PhD (plus many other letters)

No you never shunned her,
And she knew you never would.
Your belief in God and
Love of man
Ensured you never could.
So you never made
That damn old quilt
To in her memory be.
Her quilt a life,
Lives yet today,
For all the world to see.
Worry not of the things
You should have done,
But delight in the things you did.
Recall the times of joy and fun
And rejoice that we are His.

Pondering for the Road

"The weak can never forgive. Forgiveness is the attribute of the strong." –
Mahatma Gandhi

My Prayer for You

My prayer for you is that you are able to forgive, if not forget what is
behind, and sincerely consider what you are being called to do. Strain if
you have to, stand if you have to, but I pray you press on!

Sustenance for the Road

Don't allow something you have done or failed to do, or something someone
else did or failed to do to you destroy your heart. Let your past sleep. Let
it sleep on the bosom of Christ.

How do you want to go forward?

_____

_____

_____

Tell your story about the battle of forgiveness at whatilearnedwhilerunning.com

9

The Last Chapter

Therefore, since we are surrounded by such a great
cloud of witnesses, let us throw off everything that
hinders and the sin that so easily entangles, and let us
run with perseverance the race marked out for us.
Hebrews 12:1

This is actually the last chapter of this book, but I have moved it up just in case you have had more than an ample helping of reading what I have written thus far, and are not planning to finish it. That's quite all right with me, but for the sake of the beauty of this verse (Hebrews 12:1), and that which I feel compelled to testify, please at least finish this chapter before you abandon the rest. This verse from Hebrews is a favorite amongst runners and non-runners alike, so it is a treasure worth finding, phrase by phrase.

A great cloud of witnesses

In our small town, Boswell, Pennsylvania, there is a great cloud of witnesses that surrounds each other in their life's race. For many residents, it's because they were born here and they plan to die here. Outsiders, however, know that there is something special recently infused here which has created a unity that they and many lifelong families attribute to a faithful transplanted couple, Mike and Muff Dunlap. It is their special story regarding running that is worth sharing. But first, some history.

Boswell typifies a western Pennsylvania coal-mining town that thrived and bustled with jobs, businesses, churches, and taverns. Then, it slowly and painfully declined after the mine closed in 1939. When Johnstown was hit with yet another devastating flood in 1977, the surrounding towns suffered long and hard, as businesses shuttered, and prosperity seemed elusive.

Because of the perseverance of lifelong residents who did not give up on the region and simply leave, and those who chose to relocate *to* the area, the fields were ripe for seeds to be planted by a youth ministry.

So in 1989, Reverend Michael Dunlap, and his wife, Muff moved to Boswell.

"Mike," as everyone (from wee little innocent, affectionate children to troubled teenagers, grieving parents, recovering addicts and the business community) knows him, worked as a minister of a local church in Boswell, Pennsylvania. He was involved with Summer's Best Two Weeks, a renowned Christian camp in the area, and instituted a modified version of the camp as a day camp for local kids, called Boswell Day Camp.

One of the members of his congregation, Dr. Kathleen Thompson*, shared with him that she felt he was meant to start a youth ministry in the area. Before long, God did indeed call him to that vision, and his wife, Muff, and two children were on board as the North Star Youth Outreach was founded in 1997, with Thompson as a founding member who worked tirelessly to help establish the organization, staff events and build relationships with teenagers. Just a tidbit of Dr. Thompson's talents include being an integral and essential person in the Baccalaureate program and the Day Camp, and she has made thousands of her coveted cinnamon buns for the Outreach. But back to the Dunlaps.

When Mike Dunlap speaks about the history of the North Star Youth Outreach (NSYO), one of the inspirations he usually includes is the eastern Pennsylvania city of Bethlehem, home to Moravian settlers in the 1700s. What he finds remarkable about Bethlehem is that there is something "different" in a good way about the community more than 250 years after it was established. At Christmastime, many visitors, both foreign and domestic, pilgrimage to see the abundant illuminated Moravian stars hanging in doorways, candles in "every window" and to witness traditional church services.

Mike's vision was that hundreds of years from the Outreach's foundation, people would notice something different about Boswell, as they do about Bethlehem, Pennsylvania.

What makes this ministry even more interesting is that Mike and his wife Muff were equally inspired by the life of George Müller, a Prussian playboy who found himself justifiably in a German prison in 1821, where he had plenty of time to take inventory of his life, finding it utterly lacking. Four years later, the turning point in his life occurred as a university student when he attended a prayer meeting in a home and was able to comprehend and accept the love of God, and soon after he dedicated his life to becoming a missionary.

In the book, *George Müller, Delighted in God,* by Roger Steer, the story is told of Muller's journey to England where he founded orphanages strictly on prayer and faith. Müller's primary goal was not to help the poor children, or for them to be *"trained up in the fear of God,"* although those were important. Instead, *"the first and primary object of the work was that God might be magnified by the fact that the orphans under my care are provided with all they need, only by prayer and faith, without anyone being asked by me or my fellow-labourers, whereby it may be seen that God is faithful still and hears prayer still."*

So without having asked anyone for a single shilling, Müller opened and built multiple orphanages, which housed, fed, clothed, and educated over ten thousand children.

Author Steer recants a beloved story regarding Müller's faith-based life from *The Adventures of Sister Abigail*, a biographical sketch about Abigail Townsend, the daughter of close family friends. In the account, Müller led young Abigail into the orphanage dining room to show her "what our Father will do." Since there was no provision for breakfast, children stood at empty place settings when Müller prayed,

'Dear Father, we thank Thee for what Thou art going to give us to eat.' Then they all heard a knock at the door. The baker stood there. 'Mr. Müller, I couldn't sleep last night. Somehow I felt you didn't have bread for breakfast, and the Lord wanted me to send you some. So I got up at two o'clock and baked some fresh bread and have brought it.' Müller thanked the baker and

praised God for his care. 'Children,' he said, 'we not only have bread, but fresh bread.' Almost immediately they heard a second knock on the door. This time it was the milkman. 'Mr. Müller, my milk cart has broken down outside the orphanage. I would like to give the children the cans of fresh milk so that I can empty the wagon and repair it.' Müller thanked the milkman and the children enjoyed their breakfast.

Strictly on prayer, nearly one million pounds was spent on the orphanages until his death in 1898, and an additional half million pounds was directed to worldwide missionary endeavors. To translate that into today's American dollars, Bloomsby reports that from 1823 through 1924, when the pound was on the gold standard, (with the exception being during the American Civil War), a pound equaled $4.86, give or take 1 percent. Over seven million dollars was raised strictly on prayer in the 1800s. On average, throughout the 1800s, most financial citations approximate that a dollar equals 20 times that today. Even to continue underestimating, those seven million dollars would equate to *140 million dollars today*!

Imagine a ministry in today's society where needs are met strictly on prayer – no fundraisers (with the exception of students raising funds for their mission trips), no pleas for giving. What you have imagined is the North Star Youth Outreach. There have been many "empty breakfast plate moments" through the seventeen years, and Mike and Muff can testify about God's provision. It's not that the Dunlaps object to ministries that fundraise. Indeed, through tithes, the Outreach even supports them. They just feel God has called them to execute the organization like George Müller.

The aforementioned Boswell Day Camp has just celebrated its 25th Anniversary and is one of the community's cornerstone events throughout the year. Children from kindergarten through eighth grade are campers placed on either the Galatian or Roman teams. Most of the camp counselors (high school and college students) have been campers themselves, and are trained in the many rigors of responsibility for the young campers. Many take a week off work to volunteer as counselors, and a considerable number of adults volunteer as well. The week culminates in a "block party" picnic (one of the best meals of summer in my opinion) attended by approximately 300 townsfolk followed by an award ceremony where each camper and helper is acknowledged!

Additionally, Dunlap has led high school students on mission trips to Haiti every other year, with domestic trips on alternating years, and his staff are actively engaged in the lives of not only high school students, but the community.

Having lived out of state for six years, it was evident when our family returned to Pennsylvania that something was *different* about Boswell, in a good way. Our children attended a private school when we returned to the area, but after attending Boswell Day Camp in 2008, they presented us with a well-articulated argument as to why they should be allowed to attend the public school, North Star.

Although we hadn't planned to transfer schools, after running and praying (and running and praying), it seemed clear that this was God's will, although we didn't quite understand why. Some said our kids would turn out terribly. After one year, it was clear they were thriving in every way and they have been in the school ever since. It has been a blessing to be engaged in the community, to watch our children flourish with so much support outside of school.

So, in 2010 it was with much trepidation the day I learned the Outreach funds were again at critically low levels. Mike had long sacrificed being the last one to get paid his $15,000 per year salary, especially when it came time to pay the other staff, including the frugal compensation Muff received for tireless meticulous administrative oversight of NSYO. He received compensation for preaching, but still they found that they were sacrificing their own financial peace of mind, and therefore changes needed to be made.

Mike gathered the board to discuss the crisis and then outline his plan of action. My worst fear was that the Outreach would be dissolved or staff would be cut. Additionally, the Outreach tithes the donations it receives, so whenever there is a need, the Outreach is there, faithfully, emotionally, physically, and financially, giving first fruits from the inflow, regardless of the financial status.

So with a large easel board, Mike presented his plan. He was going to *eliminate* his salary altogether and take a part-time preaching position to earn the difference needed. His solution was that 100 percent of his salary would be erased from the budget.

Can you imagine any of the executives in the financial crisis that same year acting sacrificially for the greater good in that way, saying something such as "I realize that our company is suffering greatly, so instead of laying off employees, eliminating positions and reducing locations, I am going to discontinue my salary for the benefit of the company in which I believe and the people we serve." Of course you can't, because we didn't hear of any such thing. In fact, media outlets revealed greedy bonuses for these executives despite taxpayer bailouts, and their companies instituted inaccurate home foreclosures of deployed military families as well as other infractions against customers.

Reverse-tithe contributors, who give away 90 percent and utilize 10 percent for personal use, are substantially generous people who achieve a goal that would be amazing to attain. But to give 100 percent is almost incomprehensible to most people. Since that crucial moment for the Outreach, God has answered many, many prayers and been faithful to blessing the ministry even more than I'm sure I know.

In the verse from Hebrews, the author writes about running a race surrounded by a great cloud of witnesses. It's like the photographer who captures your photo during the race while encouraging you. Witnesses who can testify for you can also strengthen you, whether you are floundering or maintaining a healthy pace. This is what the Dunlaps and the North Star Youth Outreach represent for so many people and organizations locally, regionally, and even globally. It didn't take hundreds of years to see a difference, and yes, depravity and struggles still exist in our community, as in every community with human flesh. But there is light in the darkness.

So, that is the history. Here is their running story. When Mike, who has been a runner for many years, prepared to run in the hugely popular, philanthropic Somerset Daily American race for worthy charities, what he didn't know was that Muff was preparing to run with him, something she had never done before. She enlisted the help of one of the female youth leaders to train her so that she would be ready for the big day. You can imagine the logistics of arranging schedules for training runs without her husband's knowledge.

With ineffable joy, Mike tells the story about his wife surprising him before the race, with his daughters, son-in-law, and grandson in a jogging stroller as well, so that they were able to run as a family. Unabashedly, he conveys what it meant to him with words, moist eyes, and a smile that cannot be wiped off his face!

What it so heartening in addition to her sacrifice, is that so many marriages fall victim to partners secretly doing things they have no business doing, whether physical or emotional infidelity, or some other unhealthy enterprise. When we invest in our marriage, "sneaking" in a "healthy" way to please our spouse, even if it's something we don't especially enjoy, we see sacrificial love demonstrated in beautiful fashion.

This is not to slam anyone who has ever done something behind a spouse's back. My husband's favorite pastime is farming, so every now and then there is a new bull or a cow added to the herd without my knowing, usually with his co-conspirator, dear friend, and now pastor, Dan Hunsberger, delighting in my discovery of said livestock on the hillside. Dan utilizes a variant of Admiral Grace Hopper's quote "It's easier to ask for forgiveness than permission."

Everyone needs a great cloud of witnesses throughout life's race. Incredibly blessed are those who share the same DNA as those in their cloud. Even more blessed are those who support one another whether they are related or not. The question is, "What type of witnesses do you have?" Who is testifying for you? If they are not part of something great, you might want to work on your cloud.

Throw off everything that hinders

According to *The New Strong's Exhaustive Concordance Of The Bible*, in the King James Version, the word for 'everything that hinders' is *weight* from the Greek word *ogkos*. The weight to which is referred that needs to be thrown off is a burden or hindrance. What is fascinating to me is that this version of 'weight' is the only time it appears. Out of nearly 60 times the word 'weight' is used in Scripture, Strong's shows the word most often used is the Hebrew word, *mishqal,* which refers to a numerically estimated measurement, customarily used to refer to weight of silver and gold, for example. But the writer of Hebrews doesn't want to merely convey a matter of mass or heaviness.

No, the writer of Hebrews wants to convey that we need to throw off a weight that *hinders*, a *burdensome* weight, an *encumbrance*. This is more than a measurable load that is merely being carried; it's a burden that is an impediment in the race. There are so many things that can sabotage our progression in life. Interferences and obstacles abound on this course.

Generally, these deterrents are considered in a negative light as well they should. Fear is one that readily comes to mind. Why? Nearly every book of the Old Testament has at least one directive to *"Fear not"* or *"Do not be afraid."* An angel of the Lord kicks off the New Testament with just this directive to Joseph in taking Mary as his wife. Humanity's inclination is towards fearfulness and God patiently reminds us over and over to 'take courage.'

Other hindrances that can thwart us include regret, shame, and guilt. We are told to throw them off for good reason. But there may be obstacles in our lives that we consider "good things" that may be hindrances that need to be thrown off as well. Perhaps that coaching position we currently possess is a barrier to what we are meant to be doing and, additionally, is actually an obstacle to someone else stepping up to the destiny they are intended to fulfill. Or our volunteer work at the church is preventing us from the relationship path God wishes for us to pursue. Only we, with the Holy Trinity's assistance, can introspectively discern what burden we need to throw off. And then there is *the sin that so easily entangles.*

And the sin that so easily entangles

When my childhood friend, Angela Grguric, and I would run barefoot through the alleys, streets and playground of our neighborhood, we inevitably would end up in her mother's kitchen, sweaty and filthy. We would cut tomatoes from the garden or dip lettuce leaves in mayonnaise and ketchup. Angela was the youngest of thirteen children and her mother, a devout Catholic, had a small impeccable kitchen I loved to be in. On the wall, a brown piece of paper had The Seven Deadly Sins scrawled in grease pencil. My eyes were inexorably drawn to the list of words: *lust, gluttony, greed, slothfulness, anger, envy, pride.* They fascinated me, and I remember on a bold day asking what they meant. "What is gluttony?" Mrs. Grguric would give short replies and then we would be shooed back outside.

No one wants to discuss sin these days. The reality is that it *entangles*. It so easily entangles. The Apostle Paul knew this and that's why one of my favorite verses is in his first chapter of his first epistle to Timothy. *Christ Jesus came into the world to save sinners of whom I am the worst. But for that very reason I was shown mercy so that in me, the worst of sinners, Christ Jesus might display his unlimited patience as an example for those who would believe on him and receive eternal life. v 15,16*

One day you are cruising along in a state of insouciance, and the next moment your foot is caught and you are flat on your face. There is no way you are going to hear a lecture from me regarding sin. All I have to say is that sin is sin. You gossip a little? You brag on Facebook? (Remember, pride is one of the things God hates according to Proverbs 8:13) One of my favorite devotional booklets until it was discontinued was from KLOVE Radio. In an excerpt from Thursday, January 22, 2009, these words struck a nerve, *"How many times do we prevent somebody's spiritual growth, or God's blessings from coming into our own lives, because we don't control what we say? Perhaps you think that compared to adultery or stealing this is no big deal? Think again: "He who guards his lips guards his life, but he who speaks rashly will come to ruin." Proverbs 13:3*

Ouch. To throw off sin that entangles requires an honest inventory of one's life much like the one George Müller completed in prison. Hopefully it doesn't require incarceration to do that. Oswald Chambers' June 1 entry in *My Utmost For His Highest* elucidates:

If the Spirit of God has given you a vision of what you are apart from the grace of God (and He only does it when His Spirit is at work), you know there is no criminal who is half so bad in actuality as you know yourself to be in possibility.

All of us are tempted. It can be a casino or pornography or a pair of Jimmy Choo shoes. First Corinthians 10:13 assures us that we won't be tempted more than we *can bear*. Not only that, but our temptation is *common to man*, so if we look at it clearly, we see we are not alone and isolated as the enemy would have us believe. Here is what can comfort us:

No temptation has seized you except what is common to man. And God is faithful; he will not let you be tempted beyond what you can bear. But when you are tempted, he will also provide a way out so that you can stand up under it.

This is exceedingly comforting to me, because I have often heard people, especially older women, say, "God doesn't give you more than you can bear." I used to think, "Really?" It seemed so untrue when people were suffering so very much. When a night nursing supervisor assigned me to carry a stillborn baby down the back steps to the morgue, it sure seemed like that baby's mom and dad were dealt a hand more than what they could bear. When a 28 year- old woman from Chicago collapsed at Stapleton Airport due to the altitude and died weeks later in the Medial ICU, despite all our attempts to keep her alive, it sure seemed like more than her momma could bear, as I could only offer a lacking embrace. It felt like more than *I* could bear, and she was only my patient. When four more young women died of various maladies, despite every heroic medical intervention attempted, in that same Medical ICU at University Hospital the winter of 1988-1989, I felt like I would come unglued. God thought these people could bear it?

So when I realized that the statement so often misquoted is absolutely positively nowhere in Scripture, yes that comforts me. But back to sin and the way out. Where does that leave us? The way out reminds me of a tunnel that has me crouched down unable to move. It is dark and constricting. Temptation is oppressive and the conditions are stifling, making it difficult to breathe. Suddenly, the ceiling lifts, and I can stand, and gasp fresh air. There is light, outside this place, but it's up to me to take the way out. So if I'm smart, I'll run. Still, to where do I throw it off so that it doesn't so easily tangle my feet again?

There is really only one place to throw off the sin that so easily tangles so that we are not trapped again. In *The Explicit Gospel*, Matt Chandler, explains that it's the cross:

...people want to get away from the shame and the blood and the guts and the horrific slaughter of Jesus Christ and focus on something else with the cross out of the margins. But the reason we do this isn't so much to rectify an imbalance but to idolatrously elevate ourselves. It's like the charismatics who want to make the day of Pentecost central to the Christian faith. Or the Calvinists who want to make TULIP central. Liberals want to make social justice the center. Fundamentalists want to make the moral behavior the

center. (Their motto is "Do, do, do," but the cross screams out "Done!") All of those things are good things, biblical things. But to make any of them the center of the Christian faith, the grounds of our hope, is to disregard the only power of salvation-the message of the cross. We end up like Indiana Jones trying to replace the treasure with a bag of sand. We think it will work, but the whole structure comes crashing down around us. Nothing runs to the center of God's kindness and severity, demonstrating his justice, his love, and his glory all at once, besides his incarnate Son's sacrifice on the scandalous cross.

So let us run.

Let us run with perseverance

Perseverance in this verse is actually derived from the Greek word *hupomone*, which means, according to *Strong's Exhaustive Concordance, cheerful or hopeful endurance, patient continuance.*

Perseverance to me is about true grit. It's about tenacity. It's about endurance to the **nth** degree. As of this writing, Laura Hillenbrand's biography about Olympic runner and World War II hero, Louis Zamperini describes perseverance better than any. Zamperini is emulated as one of America's truest heroes in the book, *Unbroken,* recently made into a movie by the same title. My prayer before I saw the movie was that the director, Angelina Jolie, would not omit what happens to the life of Louis after he returns home from the war and recalls the promise he made to God when he was floating on a raft during a seemingly insurmountable time period when he had an epiphany and promised to dedicate his life to Him if he would not perish. ** Without spoiling the book, which you should read immediately, he indeed survives the raft only to face Japanese prison camps that make the raft look like an easy feat.

He survives and returns home to a life spiraling out of control and completely off-course. Ironically, his life's purpose post-war occurs when he finally allows himself to be "broken." It happened during a Billy Graham crusade in California, and Louis radically redirects his life's path. And, as Robert Frost concludes his notorious poem, *"And that has made all the difference."*

Louis Zamperini is one of the greatest men who has ever lived amongst the "Greatest Generation", but for all he achieved, for all he *persevered,* for all his *hopeful endurance,* it was his life and dedication after that Billy Graham crusade that defined Louis if you research this man. He dedicated his entire life to helping young kids who got into trouble just like he did as a youth. His life, in anonymity, is what I believe will earn him the words, "Well done, good and faithful servant," on the other side of heaven far more than what he achieved in his exceptional running ability, survival intrepidness, or any other valor on his part. He ran with hupomone.

This is the same *hupomone*, in Romans 15:5 for the word *endurance* in the NIV, which states, *May the God who gives endurance and encouragement give you a spirit of unity among yourselves as you follow Christ Jesus, so that with one heart and mouth you may glorify the God and Father of our Lord Jesus Christ.*

What a beautiful thing together, endurance and encouragement. Oxford Dictionary defines endurance as '*the ability to suffer patiently and without complaining or to tolerate a difficult situation for a long time.*' No wonder training in running is referred to as *increasing endurance* and marathon races are considered *endurance* events.

Certainly, running long distances requires a great deal of physical self-discipline. But most will tell you that the greater battle is within the mind, and that's where encouragement comes in.

According to *Barron's Dictionary*, the word, encourage, means to give confidence or hope; to persuade, urge, stimulate.

My husband and I were both raised in Brady Bunch families with three boys and three girls, so we have similar childhood stories that make us laugh hysterically while our only-child friends stare in horror. For example, the youngest in both families were girls, and both of our baby sisters fell out of pick-up trucks and were left behind on a family outing: his sister in Hershey, Pennsylvania and my baby sister on a Christmas tree outing in Irwin, Pennsylvania. The near-death stories really get the siblings laughing, and our mothers not, even though we somehow survived. His best family-choking story involved the boys catching glow-in-the-dark super balls bounced off the ceiling into their mouths. Mine involved marbles and spaghetti.

Stories involving our fathers are without a doubt the best. My favorite involving running comes from my in-laws. Jim's dad was a Pennsylvania State Trooper and had a chin-up bar just off the kitchen. He used to boost one of the kids up to the bar and when said child grabbed on and hung there, Jim Senior would run around the kitchen table, counting the number of times, as the mark. Davey, the middle brother, was placed on said bar and clung to it one day when they (he clinging and his father running around the table) were "going for the record." As the story is told, Davey was exclaiming that he couldn't hang on any longer when his dad encouraged him for one more lap. Davey fell and broke his nose. Jim's siblings laugh in an uproar when this story is retold, especially as their mother's face recalls it as if were yesterday. According to family legend, she wielded her maternal power as she rarely did and Dad took a saw to the chin-up bar. In family lore, there is always more laughter as the last detail is recalled. (If you can believe it, there is even a better story, with Dad the hero).

Our fathers did their best to encourage us, but thankfully we have a heavenly Father who gives us confidence and hope. *He* urges us to tolerate difficult situations for a long time! And if that weren't beautiful enough, he also gives us a spirit of unity amongst ourselves.

The problem with the human condition is that we're just too self-reliant to embrace a spirit of unity. I am the classic offender, but when my mind recalls the 1998 Great Aloha Run in Hawaii, when my husband pushed our baby, Paul, in a jogging stroller, the headline in the paper stated it perfectly: ***23,000 Feel the Love.***

We need to think of life as "race day" and we need to draw on God's gifts of endurance and encouragement to promote unity within this very difficult life. So, may the God who gives *cheerful endurance, patient continuance,* and not only that, but ***encouragement,*** give you a spirit of ***unity***. Now who would not love that?

There is another side to hupomone to consider that most are not eager to encounter. It is the word James uses to write the following:

Consider it pure joy, my brothers, whenever you face trials of many kinds, because you know that the testing of your faith develops perseverance. Perseverance must finish its work so that you may be mature and complete, not lacking anything. James 1:3,4

Colleen Tretter

Now this running with perseverance is harder to love, especially because it doesn't say, "if you face trials," but, "whenever you face trials." Truth be told, we know life has trials and through those trials, many of us do not have a cheerful endurance; we don't want our faith tested. As ordeals are prolonged, however, we can become mature and complete. Considering it pure joy is another story, and one we'll revisit in the strength-training chapter. So all that is left is the race marked out for us.

The race marked out for us.

So out of the treasure trove that is Hebrews 12:1, all that remains to address is *the race marked out for us.* Naturally, this is our life's journey; this is the course that challenges us to go the distance.

When races are marked out for us properly, there are normally arrows painted on the pavement; signs, and boundaries are clearly marked by wooden horses, for example. Race officials also help us to navigate our way. When a course omits an important directional arrow, a runner ignores it, or loses sight of runners leading the way, it is easy to head in the wrong direction. My husband and I did just that during the Hot Chocolate Run in New York one winter. We found our way back, but also discovered that others followed our errant direction, and we all ended up with a longer distance than we would have if we had stayed on course.

Just recently, over Memorial Day weekend, my son and I ran in the half marathon commemorating the 125th Johnstown Flood Anniversary, following the path of the flood. A runner ahead was shouting for us to go straight at a juncture transitioning from forest to town, so those following behind started following her. Suddenly, police officers shouted for us to travel in the direction we hadn't taken.

When we get off course in a race we can lead others astray, or be led astray. Sometimes it takes longer to get to our destination, or we can be disqualified for not staying on the route. So it is with life.

In the Book of Acts, Luke records how Paul kept his life on course as he bids farewell to the elders of Ephesus:

I only know that in every city the Holy Spirit warns me that prison and hardships are facing me. However, I consider my life worth nothing to me if only I may finish the race and complete the task the Lord Jesus has given me — the task of testifying to the gospel of God's grace. Acts 21:23,24

Paul just wants to finish the race. As a highly educated scholar, Paul would have known that Solomon, the wisest, most powerful and affluent king in the history of Israel tells us in Ecclesiastes 9:11 that,

The race is not to the swift.

Paul seems to know the fastest runner doesn't always finish the race. When my husband was in medical school, each Friday he had at least two or three exams, and he equated each one in terms of difficulty to the most challenging final exam he had the entire four years as an undergrad. It was very stressful, and he never was content with the amount of time he had to study for the end of the week, or for his performance on the exams. I don't remember who pulled him aside and asked him the question, "What do you call the person who graduates last in the class in medical school?" Jim hadn't expected the answer, "Doctor. You call him doctor, just like the first in the class." After that, he wasn't quite as anxious for those tests.

The one who completes the course marked out is a finisher, no matter how swiftly one runs. A *finisher* finishes the race. Since Hebrews 12:1 says the race *is* marked out for us (my emphasis), the implication is that there are ways to stay upon the course, allowing us to finish faster. This also implies there are ways to get off the course as well.

When I traveled with the North Star Youth Outreach to Jamaica in 2012, Mike Dunlap led a group of teenagers on afternoon runs after the workday. Running in Jamaica means in order to run towards traffic, one has to run on the right hand side of the road, rather than the left. Stepping off the curb, you have to remember to look right rather than left.

Our Jamaican driver for the trip, Vince Birthright, expertly negotiated the very bumpy road to the Jamaica Christian School for the Deaf where we were adding a second floor of classrooms to the campus, was equally adept driving through city traffic to Blossom Orphanage, where we helped with the infants and roof work. He delighted our team with this saying, "The left side is the right side, and the right side is the right side. But to drive on the right side is suicide."

While running we tried to repeat Vince's words, because it was noticeable to others in the group (and myself) that I tended to drift towards the wrong side of the road, and would veer into others, bumping them, until a busy road with a raised sidewalk kept me in check. Thankfully, my son only ran one of the days, so I only had to hear his profuse reprimands as I bumped into him just the first day.

The next day, we visited the orphanage, and as I held a tiny baby girl in my arms, I imagined how I could take her home with me. She was so little, she could surely fit into my bag, but I couldn't work out how to get her through the airport. I realized my heart was veering, just as screams from the toddler section filled the orphanage. It was bath time and I couldn't understand why there were shrieks. My philosophy in raising children (at least 50 percent of them because I only have boys) is that when they are cranky, put them in water. When they are gassy, put them in water. Perhaps this is due to the fact that my indoctrination to motherhood occurred with a five week-old in Hawaii. After my twins were born in the 'Land of Aloha' they were in water *a lot.*

So as the teenage girls held the babies, I made my way back to ask the Mennonite mission staffers what was going on and learned that there was no hot water, so the toddlers were bathed in cold water, which explained the shrieking. The hair on my neck was standing even before the next blood-curdling scream. There are no words to describe how I felt when the flash of how happy my boys were as toddlers running naked after a warm bath merged with the reality of these miserable two and three-year olds.

Also, the head caregiver tried to make us put the babies down so that they wouldn't be "spoiled" from being held. I had read enough about orphanages where babies were deprived of human touch in places like North Korea, with irrevocable implications, to challenge her and to tell the girls that if they wanted to hold the babies, to hold the babies.

The next night, after the second half of our team had spent the day at the orphanage, while the rest of us headed to the school, one of the senior girls, who had hearing issues as a young child before having a cochlear implant, came to my room sobbing. She wanted to know, "Where is God in all this?" Our first day we had been unified at the Jamaica Christian School for the Deaf, but even that was difficult as the director explained some of the children who came to be educated there were referred to as "dummy boys and dummy girls in their villages." Some had never seen a bed or indoor plumbing. Here, they had clean uniforms, food, and an education. But this day, she was at the orphanage, and sat on a hillside holding an little orphan overlooking the water with cruise ships in the distance, as I had done the day before.

While this precious girl wept on my bed, all I could do was to speak truth to her. "Where is God in all this? I absolutely positively see God in all this! We were supposed to be in Haiti in April, and when that fell through, we had no idea where we would go, but God led us to Jamaica in March. He knew that there were babies who needed to be held yesterday and today, and we had just enough arms to hold every one. They may have not fallen asleep to the sound of a human heartbeat since they were in their mothers' wombs. But yesterday and today, they were nestled with love."

The point of this story is that sometimes we are on the exact course we are meant to be on. Other times, we are veering off course as I did with my desire and ensuing plot to *steal a baby*.

More than likely, as I have done, veering off course and finding your way back from time to time is not so unusual. The second verse of Hebrews 12 advises how to run the race marked out for us, and it's something the apostle Peter could confirm from the time when he walked on water, looked at the wind and the waves, and fell under…

> *Let us fix our eyes on Jesus, the author and*
> *perfecter of our faith… Hebrews 12:2*

There are so many distractions in life that can take our focus just for a fraction of a second and cause us to sink or to veer off course. May we, like Paul, consider our life worth nothing if only we may finish the race.

Pondering for the Road

This was a long chapter and decidedly enough to mull over on the road. Hopefully the foremost thought you ponder isn't, "Why am I even reading this book?" But back to my questions in an earlier chapter, "What type of witnesses do you have?" Who is testifying for you? If they are not part of something great, you might want to work on your cloud.

My Prayer for You (even if you are thinking that)

My prayer for you is that you are not entangled in sin and that you are able to throw off every hindrance so that you may run the race marked out for YOU and only YOU.

Sustenance for the Road

As you know, we consider blessed those who have persevered. James 5:11

How do you want to go forward?

_____

_____

_____

What do you have to say about witnesses, hindrances, sin, perseverance, or the race marked out for you? Share it at whatilearnedwhilerunning.com

*An entire book could also be written about Dr. Thompson and her husband, Dr. Bill Thompson, a physician who chose to serve an area in need of medical care, and the years they have dedicated to, and sacrificed for the community of Boswell. Through teaching, coaching, serving as the physician on the sidelines…the list is endless and could never do justice to their faithful service. Kathy Thompson may have a PHD, may teach college courses, but because of her cinnamon buns, she gets to hear over and over the joke that most certainly got old years ago, "There are no buns like Dr. Thompson's buns."

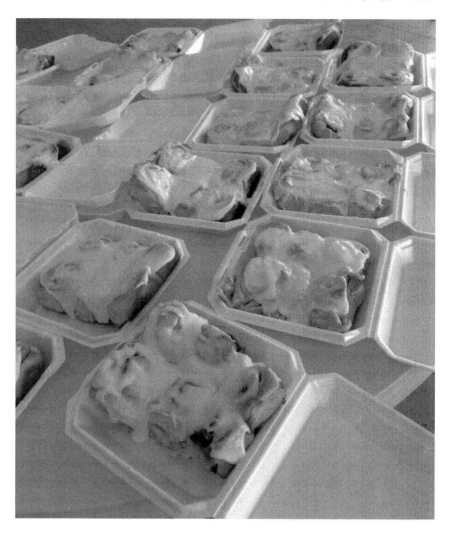

**Angelina Jolie did such a fantastic job with the movie and does indeed mention the life Louis Zamperini led in keeping with his promise to God at the end of the movie. The movie was so well done I wish she had made three movies about the book to include all that could have been told about his story! And I personally think she deserved to be nominated for an Academy Award, even though I was not one of her biggest fans prior to the movie. Not that anyone cares what I think about that, but still I just had to testify as a witness for her.

10

Running Downhill Isn't All It's Cracked Up To Be

I lift my eyes to the hills-
where does my help come from?
My help comes from the LORD,
the maker of heaven and earth.
Psalm 121:1,2

If you have continued to read after the "Last Chapter," hopefully you are not feeling adverse stress from persevering on this journey with me. No one wants trials in this life. We want to cruise downhill in relative ease. We want to be happy, healthy, and prosperous. We don't want stress, yet many people are still very stressed in a negative way. You don't have to search the topic of stress and health while your stress relief candle burns nearby, or review American Psychology Association articles while you squeeze a stress relief ball to know that truth. An Internet search of *stress relief products* yields over 5 million results. So if we know that living in a state of stress is detrimental to one's health, why are so many of us doing so? The fact is that we *do* need a certain amount of stress to be healthy, whether we are completing an important college application deadline or reporting to work on time.

Eustress (yoo 'stres) is a term that refers to positive stress according to the Gale Encyclopedia of Medicine. This does not refer to an absence of stress. We just aren't meant to plop on the couch and watch every hour of the Today Show followed by Kelli and Michael, followed by Ellen, followed by – you get the picture. Now don't get me wrong. It's not wrong to catch your favorite show, or more than a few of them. A college student just finishing the rigors of finals might just need a *Lost* marathon to decompress, so it's not the actual *viewing* that can be a problem, but when that is all someone does, living in a state of so little stress, day in and day out; it is in fact *stressful*. It's a lot like running downhill.

Running downhill feels wonderful. You can catch your breath, go faster without much effort, and let gravity do the work. Just stretch out your legs and go. However, when you run downhill for a long time, well then it's not all it's cracked up to be, and it's a lesson that is learned easily when you live in a mountainous region, and one I learned in the early 1990s while training for my first marathon and running in my second.

The Johnstown YMCA Marathon begins at the top of the World's Steepest Vehicular Inclined Plane. Beginning at the top of the vista overlooking the Johnstown valley that multitudes of floods had impacted, the race route winds through one of my favorite cathedral tree lines in the Continental United States (Luzerne Street) eventually to the apex of Saint Clair Road. Saint Clair Road top to bottom is over two miles downhill. Cars are not too big a problem on this thoroughfare, so it's still worth traveling down, but it's a loonnnngg way down. It seems like a great route especially since it's the road traveled in the actual marathon before heading up one side of the Conemaugh River Gap via Route 56 (West) and enjoying the view of the gorge on the way back down 403 (South).

After running down Saint Clair Road a few times, I notice my toes are starting to hurt, especially the middle toes in particular despite having shoes designed with wide toe boxes. The downhill pounding also seems to affect my knees, and I have to be conscientious about how my feet plant, because I have had a few scares too many with my ankles turning, and when I stumble, it is a sprawling, flailing mess, taking more than a few moments to gain purchase of solid ground. Come to think of it, as I catch myself, "what is that in the ditch?" I see trash I never saw running uphill. What a mess! After the runs, my knees are so stiff I can barely get down on them to test the bath water for a long soak. Then, within days my toenails are discolored, and I mean in an unattractive dark purplish-black way. The Emergency Department physicians with whom

I work now tell me I can kiss them goodbye, because they are goners. Not long after the marathon, my toenails fall off as I was told they would. So I realize running downhill is not all it's cracked up to be.

Have you ever noticed that when life is going along relatively easy, you negatively react to something that is insignificant on a global scale? Most of us in the United States are relatively healthy and prosperous when compared to the remainder of the world's population. In fact, according to a 2013 Gallup report of 131 countries and regions, median annual household incomes worldwide are $9,733. Furthermore, the top 10 wealthiest populations report that the median per capita incomes are *fifty times* those of the poorest 10 populations. However, if you compare an average person from Liberia, who was at the bottom of the list at $118 per capita income with an average person from the United States, with an average of $15,480, you see the number is *131 times.* In a worldwide comparison, prosperity most definitely does exist in the United States.

Regarding health, while I was working as a nurse in that Emergency Department, there was not a child who required an antibiotic or pain medication who was denied. Without intending to offend anyone, even if a parent had two packs of cigarettes in their purse, but claimed they couldn't afford to fill the antibiotic prescription, we provided it for them, for the sake of their child. It really rankled some staff members, but didn't matter to me. Imagine being a parent who has no medication to lower a child's fever. No Tylenol. No Ibuprofen. That is the rest of the world. A baby born with a cleft lip in the United States has it repaired almost immediately. Watch a Smile Train infomercial to see how it impacts children on the rest of the planet.

I'm not saying we don't have real illnesses or suffer, because we do, but we take for granted what is available to us. Comparatively speaking, we are cruising downhill and we aren't happy. Our toenails are turning black and blue. The icemaker isn't working, bills are tight and the car needs new breaks. We are stressed. We see the trash on the side of the road.

Carrying the kitchen trash bag as I do most every month to clean the trash on our road at the end of a run, I jog and grab. When you adopt a road it's like adopting a turtle. As my sister Lisa told me, "Before you get it you need to decide who gets it in your will – and be glad you're dead." (That was regarding the turtle, not the road ☺.) As part of a cleanup program, the expectation is that the road will be cleaned twice yearly, usually in the spring and fall. The trash that gets discarded on our road requires monthly maintenance. Cleaning a road also requires a lot of forgiveness, because the same offenders toss the same items. At first I have compassion on the litterbug ruffians, because presumably they are all illiterate. Every item I pick up has in bold print capital letters, **DO NOT LITTER**. However, after picking up the two-picante sauce opened packets with the Taco Bell burrito wrappers for the twentieth time, I want the offender to **not** 'Live Más.' I especially despise the double cheeseburger wrappers-large fries containers and McDonald's bag strewn across the road each evening around 8 pm. I am becoming a trash connoisseur of cans of cheap beer and energy drinks.

Qualifying the worst things to pick up supersedes quantifying the number of items. You would think a used diaper, a hypodermic needle, or five laundry detergent containers filled with motor oil would be the worst thing to clean. But you would be wrong. The worst thing to clean isn't even the empty animal feedbag that I came across which had been used for an emergency bowel movement by some poor farmer. He must have had a long day in the tractor. No, the most profane item I had to clean knocked the wind out of me the second I spotted it. It was similar to the feeling I had when I was seven or eight years old and ran full speed into a glass door at a hotel where we were staying. I was launched backwards at least five feet and left breathless. The litter on the ground was a Happy Meal box. In an instant, I pictured a child in the backseat of a car with safety windows that only go down so far watching as their parent tosses the box out the front window. And a new generation of litter hooligans is born, leaving me apoplectic and exasperated.

If you're like me, you can be consumed by something so trivial like the trash on the side of a road. But then a real challenge arises, which puts it all into perspective. A child is hurt; an ambulance ride and a trip to the operating room and suddenly nothing else matters except "I need help." I forget about the trash. Suddenly I am looking up for a break in the treacherous storm forming around me.

I lift my eyes to the hills-
where does my help come from?
my help comes from the LORD
the maker of heaven and earth. Psalm 121:1,2

We don't just rise to the occasion on our own; we seek God in times of crisis. When I run one of my usual routes these days, there is an uphill climb that lasts approximately 1.5 miles. It's difficult and easy to get out of breath unless a distinct effort is made to control breathing in the way I was taught in gym class: in through the nose, out through the mouth. Utilizing arm motion is essential to making the ascent in conjunction with a concentrated exertion in stride. I look up and see the sky and treetops and my face lifts to the splash of sunshine through the trees. My toenails don't fall off and my knees don't hurt. When I stumble, I regain my footing much easier than on a downhill run.

July 2002. As I returned from my route, I cooled down by walking the nearly half mile trek up our farm lane. I saw my neighbor, Dale on the bulldozer clearing the brush and overgrowth from our hillside. Palpable concern for his welfare as he cruised up the steep hills of our acreage paled in comparison to the anguish everyone in the community was feeling as nine miners were trapped underground in the Quecreek Mine, 10 miles south of us. Dale's friend, one of the miners, causes deep concern for him on a personal level. I only learned of the accident two mornings previously at the Vacation Bible School the kids were attending, but the miners have been trapped since Wednesday evening. Prayers for the men and their families popped up on restaurant signs, in emails, and were lifted at every opportunity during the ecumenical VBS (Episcopal, Presbyterian, United Church of Christ, Church of the Brethren). It seemed everyone in the county was praying, and as television stations kept vigil, the nation was watching, too.

We lift our eyes to the hills. *As a family, we were supposed to go on vacation Sunday to Stone Harbor, New Jersey, but I was afraid that even if the miners survive, some of them would require amputations of their fingers and toes at least, because of the cold water in that mine that trapped them. I told my husband, one of the few vascular surgeons Board Certified to do amputations, "that is a lot of fingers and toes." So we planned to leave Monday, because we should know the outcome by Sunday.*

Where does our help come from? *There were numerous roller-coaster-like reports that caused optimism, from the sound of banging nine times which indicated all 9 miners were alive to negative news of problems with the drilling progress, and then a miracle in how the right equipment showed up at just the right time.**

Our help comes from the LORD. *The families were gathered at the Sipesville Fire Hall, and some at the actual rescue site. Many hearts ached for the agony they were enduring. The rescuers went without sleep. Even the young fireman who was managing traffic on Route 985 when we left Somerset Thursday was still there Friday morning. When we drove by, I offered him coffee and donuts, but he told me there was food at the fire hall.*

The maker of heaven and earth. *We know as a community that this could end badly. We lived through it when the plane crashed nearby in Shanksville on 9/11. Some people are sure the miners won't survive. Others would never entertain such a thought. It is all anyone was talking about. As I finished walking up our lane, I suspected the community would come together just as it did ten months previously on September 11, 2001. The pastors told the children at VBS that they know the Lord will help us through regardless of an outcome no one can predict, but oh, we pray earnestly for the survival of these men and their families. Overnight, the world watches as miner after miner is raised in that yellow rescue basket, healthier than anyone could have expected! The rejoicing of the miracle Sunday morning across the County was palpable. It was beyond glorious, almost incomprehensible the joy and celebration that ensued!*

We should not forget these times of wonder in our lives but we do. If only the emotion and memory could stay as fresh as the day of rejoicing, but the next thing you know, we're complaining about the weather or griping about the cost of bananas. The truth of it according to James is that, *"We all stumble in many ways." James 3:2* How do we stumble? Well, he tells us in the very next verse: *If anyone is never at fault in what he says, he is a perfect man, able to keep his whole body in check. James 3:3* Our tongues are the problem. Our worst stumbling comes from the words we say, so much so that half of the chapter is about taming the tongue, but James admits no man can tame it (verse 8). Yes, in many ways we stumble, as I learned after a run with my husband when he was stationed in Hawaii.

Jim's parents arrived for their month-long visit as they did every February since we moved to Hawaii. They offered to babysit the three boys so that we could have a couple nights away. We flew to the nearest island, Molokai, made famous by Father Damien's work at the leper colony, and stayed at the 56,000-acre Molokai Ranch in a tentalow next to the ocean.

Being able to sleep through the night was heavenly. Whales were in abundance off shore, and we took advantage of the freedom and went on a nice long run along a secluded path that emerged on the beach and we came upon a large green sea turtle. It was paradise. Even though our bodies weren't used to it, we also biked about 8 miles from the lodge to the pavilion where food was available. Jack Hanna, the veterinarian zookeeper, and his crew from his television show on animal adventures were there to film the whales that week. When we walked into the pavilion in our still somewhat sleep-deprived, famished state, spent from our adventures, the menu on the dry erase board began like this:

Kona Coffee
Herbal Tea
Whale Milk
Fresh fruit...

Before I could process in my brain that there was actually an "O" in Whole, and that it was just the way someone hastily wrote the letter so that it looked like an "A", I exclaimed to my husband in front of Jack Hanna's crew, "Look! They have whale milk!" As soon as I said it, I froze, he froze, the crew froze, and when I slowly turned to look my husband in the eye, we both just exploded with laughter! For the remainder of the trip, and every time we saw Jack Hanna on television thereafter, my husband would occasionally break into a demonstration of the motion utilized for milking cows. Oh how we laughed. Boy did I stumble in it that day with my tongue! It can be much, much worse, though. That could be qualified as a stumbling uphill moment, but we have all certainly had stumbling downhill moments: flailing-can't-catch-ourselves-heart-stopping messes in what we say, which is why we must remember what James says in the first chapter: If anyone considers himself religious and yet does not keep a tight rein on his tongue, he deceives himself and his religion is worthless. (James 1:26) Hopefully someone out there can say "yikes!" with me.

Lastly, one of the many ways in which we stumble in what we say is completely accidental because the words we speak are not the words we wish for the listener to hear. Word for word, they are accurate. Alas, an inflection here or a pause there, and our stumbles in being misconstrued are complete. For example, one of my sister's friends was having problems with her houseplants, and she complained to the nursery worker that she thought they were dying from over-watering. He showed her the lovely fuchsia hanging baskets that are so often for sale in May. She adored the flowering plant, but when he stated, "You can't give these **too much** water!" she heard the admonishment, "You **can't** give these too much water." When my sister saw her dried up dead hanging baskets, she figured out what her friend had misinterpreted. It still makes me chuckle.

The words were correct; the interpretation not so much, and these were spoken face to face. Add email, texting, and social media to the mix and it's no wonder as to why we are stumbling in so many ways with the words we don't even speak but *type*.

Stumbling on this arduous journey called life should be a reminder to look no further than *the* place for help, but it can be easier said than done. Sometimes it takes facing a mountain that is daunting and beyond the human capacity perceived to ascend. For Moses, that mountain led to an encounter with God, but it took going the distance to the burning bush. (Exodus 3). For Peter, James and John, that ascent led to witnessing the transfiguration. (Luke 9:8-36). Even after getting to the top of a hill, we may be called to dig down to our reserves and overturn tables in righteous anger as Jesus did at the Temple Mount. (Matthew 21:12-17).

My own personal hills bring new insight and wisdom, but as I look up to the Maker of heaven and earth, I am reminded that my knees aren't so stiff so that I can't bend them. Indeed, this is the very best place to be as the words of the very wise pastor of In Touch Ministries, Dr. Charles Stanley teaches, "Fight your battles on your knees."

So the next time an insurmountable climb is before you, remember you may just discover your own burning bush with all ten toenails intact.

Pondering for the Road

When was the last time you lifted your eyes to the hills? Great peace have they who love your law, and nothing can make them stumble. Psalm 119:165

My Prayer for You

My prayer for you is to realize, without condemnation, how you stumble, intentionally or unintentionally, and that your stumbling block can then be removed.

Sustenance for the Road

Listen to the song Praise You In This Storm *by Casting Crowns*

How do you want to go forward?

_____

_____

_____

Do you have an experience to share regarding the hills of life? Share it at whatilearnedwhilerunning.com.

* If you don't believe in miracles anymore, visit the Quecreek Mine Rescue site. I had the opportunity to travel to Haiti in 2013 on the same mission team as Bill Arnold, landowner (along with his wife, Lori) of Dormel Farms, where the mine rescue occurred. He retold the story of those fateful few days from the first knock on his door late Wednesday evening to the miracle of the rescue with the clarity and emotion that only someone who experienced it firsthand can. He knows a miracle happened on his land and he and his wife have dedicated themselves to testifying about it with a museum and historical articles from the rescue. If you ever visit PA, check it out

Colleen Tretter

11

Hydration: Living Water

Take me to the river, drop me in the water
Take me to the river, dip me in the water.
~Talking Heads song

He will lead them to springs of living water.
And God will wipe away every tear from their eyes.
Revelation 8:17

You might be wondering how it is that the second-most vital requirement for life sustenance (after air) could be so far down the list of lessons learned so I implore you to believe that this position is no reflection upon the extent to which water is cherished by me. Perhaps the very essential nature of water is why I find it so difficult to convey the preciousness of hydration while running.

The quintessential simplicity of hydration was evident in the 1980s when I started running long distances in that A) you became thirsty and so B) you quenched your thirst with water. That's it. A and B. Thirsty? Drink! Then the message to be learned was that the time to drink is *before* getting thirsty. Before you get thirsty: drink! During Penn State ROTC exercises, the nurse cadets conveyed the message to other cadets to "pee pale."

In the 1990's, devices were made so that you could carry water in packs around your waist as you ran, and you could drink from a long plastic straw. Electrolyte replacement drinks came on the market and an entire strategy seemed to revolve around utilizing them, especially during long races. Next, the explosion of bottled water hit the market and it seemed no one should be able to live, even if they weren't running, without at least 6 bottles a day! You can buy a case of 24 bottles for approximately $5, but every concession stand sells them for minimally $1 a bottle. As an aside, wouldn't you just fall over if you were charged twenty cents for a bottle of water? When we were at a Mumford and Sons concert recently, we waited in line for water, and when we got to the front of the line, they were charging *four dollars*. I asked the poor guy who waited on me if that was for a case or a bottle; he was not amused.

So I regret to say that as time has gone by, I have not kept up with the twists and turns of hydration. With each passing year, however, I appreciate this resource more. Having no water for things other than drinking for even a day is so inconvenient for most people, that it cannot be ignored; whether for cooking, bathing, washing clothes and dishes, or watering plants. Recent droughts throughout the country surely make people cherish water.

It is still astonishing to me that the same substance that quenches your thirst and cools your body when you sweat it through your pores, makes crops grow, and is something that when heated, provides muscle relief after running. Whether a warm bath, steam shower, or a hot tub, the water is deliciously wonderful. Furthermore, you can add salts or special soaks for added relief. Even a dip in a pool after a long run is gloriously refreshing.

Then, when you twist your ankle or have a sore knee, the identical molecule in the form of ice provides one of the most important therapeutic measures you can utilize. My children know that one of my first questions when they are injured is, "Did you put ice on it?"

And then there's snow. Although I'm a huge proponent of wearing bright clothing while running outside, I'm a fan of black gloves for the sheer reason that when it starts to snow, you can sometimes see the myriad of crystalline shapes as the flakes land on your hands. I never tire of delighting in examining the delicate structures, perhaps because they are impermanent. Elusive or not, if the chemicals in my body could be measured when snowflakes land on my gloves, they could cure something I'm sure. Runners who appreciate snow, because they are usually fit, don't have to be children to enjoy the white stuff as it accumulates to sled ride, ski, or build snowmen, and it's all thanks to water.

Water is also widely touted as beneficial for those who are concerned about the effects of aging. Time for a confession. Remember when I stated that in the *My Big Fat Greek Wedding* of life, running is the Windex? Well, when it comes to wrinkles, maybe not so much, but then again my complexion comes from my fair and freckled Irish heritage. Because I prefer to run outside regardless of weather, the summer sun and cold winter winds have taken their toll over the past thirty years; I have earned my wrinkles. * I once had numerous invitations from mothers of my children's' classmates to anti-aging skin product parties, and never had time to attend. Finally, one of the moms just dropped off the sample kit. God love her because heaven knows she tried to help me look better. Unfortunately, I was already fifteen years older than most of those moms. In my family, the joke is that the good news is that when you're 40, you have a pretty good idea how you are going to look at 60; the bad news is that when you're 40, you like you're 60! My eldest brother used this to his advantage on the tennis court when facing youngsters; they never anticipated a killer left-hand serve from the old geezer.

The truth is that well-hydrated skin does lead to a more youthful appearance. According to a 2010 study in the British Journal of Dermatology, an average 28-year-old woman with dry skin had a 52% increase in wrinkles by the age of 36, but only a 22% increase with well hydrated skin. So if you must run outside, wear sunscreen, use moisturizers and drink water. For some women, having fewer wrinkles is reason enough to consider water's importance to survival second only to air.

All of the previous illustrations are just a few examples of how an essential substance to life can also bring healing and delight, and recreation involving ponds, lakes, rivers and oceans has not even been addressed! No wonder *the Spirit of God was hovering over the waters* in the second verse of the Holy Bible (Genesis 1).

Noah built an ark to survive it (Genesis 7), Moses parted it (Exodus 14), John baptized with it (John 1), Jesus made wine with it (John 2), then He walked on it (Matthew 14), calmed a storm of it with just a rebuke (Mark 4), and woke up a woman at the well by teaching about it in the form of living water (John 4). Although the last example isn't considered to be a miracle, for that woman I believe it was. Sometimes a splash in the face changes everything.

My literal splash in the face came in 1984, when my brother convinced me to be his partner and to attempt to dance in the Penn State Dance Marathon, after his coworker and his coworker's partner had to withdraw just days before because of an injury. The coveted reserved spot was just one of 500 for the couples who wanted to participate in the 48-hour event known as THON. It was (and still is) the largest student-run philanthropic event in the world benefitting the Four Diamonds Fund for kids with cancer. Beginning at 7pm on Friday through 7pm Sunday, we were going to dance. Although I reminded my brother of my notoriously pathetic ability to stay up late just for even one night, he was convinced we could do it. So when we turned up and were asked for our team name, we gave them "Bob and Stacy" so that the money they had raised could be contributed. We collected the shirts that had been reserved for Bob and Stacy, and then started dancing! Every eight hours, we had a three-minute break to run to the bathroom, run back to the gym and dive on mats where morale volunteers massaged our aching feet.

*I held up surprisingly well until Sunday morning, after the crowd of onlookers, the "bar crowd," who had arrived after the bars closed at 2 am, came and went home. My detachment from reality came on like a fog, and I distinctly recall my agitation and the dismay on my brother's face when I grabbed his shirt and insisted that there was a conspiracy to confuse us and that the walls had been switched and that there was a pit in the middle of the floor. "And they keep calling me Stacy!" (I was wearing Stacy's shirt with her name on the back.) He was discussing with our friends who were also dancing what to do with me, and I remember hearing the words, "dropping out" used. Somehow I made my way to a trashcan filled with melting ice and when I splashed it on my face multiple times, something brought me back from the abyss. ***

Yes, water is of staggering importance. When water is unsafe for drinking in the United States, boil notices make the news. Water distribution centers are set in place. So when you travel to a country where the water is so precarious that it's not even safe to brush your teeth with it, it is distinctly noticeable. Because water is so essential, inhabitants will use it as long as they can access it, regardless of risk.

The first time I passed by a river outside of Port au Prince, Haiti filled with trash and debris – even a rusty vehicle and animal carcass – where a mass of humanity was washing clothes, bathing, eliminating (mostly half-naked children), and scooping water to be hauled on shoulders, the image was forever imbedded in my mind. This is the reality for much of the world. Perhaps this is why this chapter is so hard to write. (Another form of fluid loss besides sweat – that is, tears – is inevitable.)

Having seen this in Port-au-Prince, Haiti, it was even more disheartening when a second pastor, Pastor St. Hillaire, was murdered after our mission trip in 2008. The anguish and emptiness so many of us felt over his death were similar to the words in Psalm 22, a psalm of despair, *I am poured out like water (verse 14)*. The grief was as physically distressing as being dehydrated and thirsty, in a parched way.

But Isaiah 55 begins with, "Come, all you who are thirsty, come to the waters...." There is a hope for those of us who thirst. It wasn't until I had the opportunity to return to Haiti with Living Hope Mission in Cap-Haitien that my grief was quenched with hope.

Living Hope Mission could have an entire book written about it, but this is my brief synopsis. Founded by Wilbert Merzilus and his wife, the mission is unique in that since the inception of the ministry, an interesting strategy is utilized to address the desperate needs of the Haitian people. Perhaps the strategy works because so many outsiders come in and try to "fix" Haiti. Wilbert describes his impoverished childhood as typical for many Haitian children. He was raised in a rural area of northern Haiti, and as he told our team with smiling eyes on the trip that was so restorative to me, he was "like one of the naked children you see" as you travel through the country. He had been helped, by being brought out of that area to attend school, and it was as if someone had reached down and pulled him out of the pit, by allowing him to be educated. Then Wilbert had a benefactor, a woman from Florida, who sponsored him to receive an education in the United States. He could have been content to remain in the States, live a comfortable life, and enjoying the relative abundance of the U.S., but he could not forget the children in Haiti. Even if he could only pull one child up at a time, he would later tell us, that as long as there were children living in such insufficiency, he felt compelled to help them.

How Living Hope did that is a model that is unique to U.S. citizens, who want to rush in and try to feed and clothe those in need. The strategy enlisted was that first, when a "church" was established, and by that I

113

mean people gathering to worship in a space, such as on a sandy lot under trees, then a well was built so that water would be available. Then an actual physical church was built, which can be a painstakingly laborious process, starting with walls, then the roof, and finally the floor. As in most third world countries, concrete is mixed by hand using buckets of gravel and bags of cement and poured bucket by bucket, generally in hot and humid conditions. Next a school was built. Then, a feeding program was established for the students who attend the school. Through twenty plus years of Living Hope Mission, there are 18 churches and 13 schools in northern Haiti. But then tragedy by way of maliciousness struck Wilbert.

Prior to the mission trip to Jamaica mentioned in Chapter 9, our team's intended destination was to be to the Living Hope Mission in Cap-Haitien, Haiti, but during our planning and fundraising in late 2011, Wilbert was kidnapped. The story he told us in person in 2013 was almost identical to what had been conveyed after the incident occurred. He was knocked unconscious, blindfolded, hands tied and thrown into a vehicle. The kidnappers called for ransom. He awoke in darkness inside the vehicle, hearing the kidnappers' voices in front of the vehicle and managed to work his blindfold so that he could see by headlights that there was water flooding the roadway, so deep that it was questionable whether they could pass.

The doors to the vehicle were open, so Wilbert worked his way out and into the brush, bleeding from his head. When the kidnappers realized he was gone from the vehicle, they searched for him, but despite some terrifying moments when they were close to where he hid in the dark, they could not locate him and left the scene. Through the night, Wilbert followed the sounds of chickens (where there are roosters, there are people), and made his way to a town he recognized and went to the home of a friend, where he then was granted aid and safety. His wife was unaware that he had escaped. Ransom had been paid. The kidnappers were eventually caught, and one of them was someone who had been helped by Living Hope.

To heal from the trauma of the incident, Wilbert took a sabbatical to the United States. Obviously, some people would recommend *not* returning to the mission, but that's what Wilbert did. He continues to pour himself out as a living sacrifice for the benefit of one child at a time.

In an amazing twist of irony, following the catastrophic earthquake, the Dominican Republic (the country that shares the island of Hispaniola) built a university geographically in the center of these Living Hope schools. So the only gap between the Living Hope schools (which typically go no further than 8th grade) and the university is the middle school (what we call high school). Wilbert's dream, and the goal of many for that continuity are coming to fruition. It is now under construction.

Some nights I dream I am back in the Living Hope compound, hearing voodoo drums in the distance, and awaken with the familiar yearning for Haiti and the proximity of such purposeful, sacrificial living.

While so many of us live like the Dead Sea, receiving, receiving receiving with no outflow, Wilbert lives like the Sea of Galilee – flowing, life-giving water in a land where it is so scarce. *Living* hope.

Isaiah 58:11 quenches my thirst and captures the guidance and comfort I need in times of dehydration of spirit. I hope it does the same for you.

The LORD will guide you always;
He will satisfy your needs in a sun-scorched land
And will strengthen your frame.
You will be like a well-watered garden,
Like a spring whose waters never fail.
Isaiah 58:11

Pondering for the Road

Are you feeling parched now and as though you are wandering in a desert? What is your oasis, or does it feel like there is none in sight? Just after the psalmist describes great suffering (I am poured out like water. Psalm 22:14), comes the Psalm with an opening line almost everyone can recite, even if they don't read scripture: The LORD is my shepherd, I shall not be in want. He makes me lie down in green pastures, he leads me beside quiet waters, he restores my soul. *(Psalm 23:1, 2) but many don't know that in verse 5…*my cup overflows.

My Prayer for You

My prayer for you is that with joy you will draw water (Isaiah 12:3) *when you need it most.*

Sustenance for the Road

As the deer pants for streams of water,
So my soul pants for you, O God.
My soul thirsts for God, for the living God.
Psalm 42:1,2

How do you want to go forward?

_____

_____

_____

Do you have a story to share regarding hydration or living water? Share it at whatilearnedwhilerunning.com.

*(In my defense, sunscreen was barely used in the 1980s; indeed some people even added a few drops of Betadine to baby oil to stimulate melanocytes for darker skin!)

** That experience of sleep-deprived hallucinating helped me tremendously as a night shift nurse when patients developed ICU psychosis or just simply had what some called "sundowner's syndrome," or simply when there was a full moon.

12

Wrong Paths Versus Right Paths

Two paths diverged in a yellow wood,
And sorry I could not travel both
And be one traveler, long I stood
And looked down one as far I could
To where it bent in the undergrowth ....
-from The Road Not Taken by Robert Frost

One of the greatest privileges with which I have been blessed has been to accompany middle school girls to summer camp, a physically grueling undertaking that could not be accomplished at my age without a baseline fitness level. We literally *run* around camp at all hours of the day and evening. One night we were sent on an obstacle course with the mission of protecting the grounds from "the elderly" (twenty-something camp staff wearing old robes and gray wigs) who were trying to "take over" the camp. As we crossed the quad, yelling and ducking water balloons, then climbing a wooden wall, the irony that *I* was the old person was not lost on me. When we raced to the path to reach the lake – our final destination – and the "elderly" jumped out waving canes, we breathlessly ***screamed*** as if they were ax murderers about to attack us! It was ludicrous fun.*

The serious (and physically restorative) side of camp involves cabin times that give remarkable insight as the girls have allowed me glimpses of their precious lives. Year after year, a prevalent desire they express comes from a version of the question, "What prayer would you like God to answer in your life if He were to clearly speak to you?" Almost unanimously, despite all other circumstances in their lives, the girls wish for discernment for their life's direction. They want to know what their purpose is in life. They want to be sure they are on the right path.

It makes my heart swell for them and feel relief that humans are not God, because if I could answer their prayers instantaneously, I would. But God loves them so much more, and even though I have shared Jeremiah 29:11 with them: *"For I know the plans I have for you,"* declares the LORD... *"plans to prosper you and not to harm you, plans to give you hope and a future,"* they still think a crystal ball would be nice. Sharing with them that my years of traveling this journey, seeking Him and finding Him, has shown me something. It has shown me that as with all of His children, He wants them to seek Him for discernment at every fork in the road, because there are countless junctures as *"way leads on to way,"* to borrow from Robert Frost's third stanza of *The Road Not Taken*. They still would like a crystal ball.

When my husband and I used to run together, I preferred paths with familiarity, to the extent that I was content if we ran halfway in one direction, then turned around and came back to the original starting place, so that I knew where we were going. Jim, however, always wanted to try a new route home, and would suggest trying a different way that we had not explored. Sometimes it would end up great and we discovered a preferable path, but often it resulted in getting slightly lost, running further than what we had planned. My crankiness would be evident when we would reach a juncture and argue about the correct way back.

As years have gone by, my belief and experience is that in this life there is not *a* fork in the road with only two choices from which to choose, but actually **four** types of paths. (It's like jogging through one of our local state parks).

Here are the four types paths I have identified thus far, but in ten years, I may find a few more.

1. Paths we are not meant to take and we know we are not meant to take them but we take them anyhow.
2. Paths we are not meant to take but we think we are meant to take them, so we do.
3. Paths we are meant to take and we know it, but we don't or won't.
4. Paths we are meant to take; we know this, and we take them regardless where they lead.

This last one is the only true and correct path upon which we ought to be, but how to know? Both Psalms and Proverbs have a lot to say about paths, as the words path, paths or pathway are mentioned thirty-three times. God has revealed much to me through the many years of literally and figuratively finding myself on each of these paths.

1. Paths we are not meant to take and we know we are not meant to take them but we take them anyhow.

Inevitably as a runner, you will encounter signs warning of danger. On the island of Kauai, Hawaii, in 1988, my husband and I encountered a sign entering the tropical forest that could not have been more clearly defined. It said

DANGER
STOP DO NOT ENTER.
SLIPPERY ROCKS AT TOP OF FALLS.
PEOPLE HAVE BEEN KILLED.
KEEP OUT.

That is the actual punctuation of the sign. Perhaps if there were more exclamation points, we would not have exercised our stupidity and kept on going. People have been KILLED!!! Keep OUT!!! Maybe that emphasis would have done the job, but regardless, we kept going. Emerging at the origin of twin beautiful waterfalls was plenty frightening so we thankfully did not venture out onto the rocks like some other daredevils have been known to do, some as their very last act.

Most of us have met people who *always* seem to make the wrong choices. It's as if they charge past every single danger sign purposefully. Some people make it a continuous pattern, despite all the warning signs, even when it requires more effort to take the wrong path than the right one. They agree to hang out with the wrong people. They go places they know they shouldn't. They know they shouldn't marry someone, but do it anyway. Having lived in close proximity to someone who succumbed to addiction in the present heroin epidemic gave a birds' eye view of one wrong path after another in this lifestyle. Every decision leads to more destruction and devastation. Regarding the wrong path, Proverbs 4:14 says, *Do not set foot on the path of the wicked or walk in the way of evil men. The path of the righteous is like the first gleam of dawn, shining ever brighter till the full light of day.*

Nevertheless, any of us can land on this path at any time, just as my husband and I did at that warning sign. The real danger holds double jeopardy when a) we think we are immune to jumping on that wrong path and b) the wrong path isn't always obviously wicked. We think we are in control but start flirting with disaster in, say a relationship, and soon we knowingly head down this wrong road. When the choice is seemingly good such as accepting a promotion or buying a house, it can still be the *wrong* path. Even more difficult is when others point us down this path and give advice about why this venture is the way we should go. "Of course you should take the job because you will get a raise." Nonetheless, these people aren't God, and no matter how important they are to us, they still may not be pointing the way to the correct route.

Psalm 119 has a lot to say about the right path and is rich with guidance as well as defining the illumination we need. *Your word is a lamp to my feet and a light to my path.* (Psalm 119:105) So the path can be lit for us, but perhaps we have not turned on the switch.

2. Paths we are not meant to take but we think we are meant to take them, so we do.

No better story exists than the multi-layered parable of the Prodigal Son to demonstrate this point. Most people know this story, and have heard it so often that they inaccurately use the term "prodigal" to describe a "favorite" son. Prodigal, however, is defined as reckless and wasteful. So this son asks his father for his inheritance so that he can set off down the road he wants. He doesn't seek his father's guidance. He doesn't ask for advice. In his selfishness, he believes this is the path he should take. His father doesn't try to stop him, and the reckless, wasteful son finds himself in a foreign land living wildly. After he has squandered all the money, he found a job feeding pigs, yet was starving and longed to eat the pig's food. Scripture tells us that he came finally to his senses, and realized his sin against his father and heaven, and in repentance, decides to ask for a position of one of his father's hired hands.

He went to his father, doubling the distance he traveled on a path he never should have taken in the first place and *while he was still a long way off, his father saw him* (Luke 15:20). What does his father do? His father *runs* to him. He doesn't stand there. He doesn't walk. While his son is still a long way off, his father *runs* to him.

Many theologians make the point that this would be inappropriate in the day. Men wore robes and sandals, so to run would require hoisting robes and revealing legs, and generally would be very undignified. But his father doesn't care. He *runs* to his son. When we head back home to God, *He runs toward us.* Even when we are still a long way off, **God runs.** When a path is before us that we think we are meant to take, we are wise to seek our Father's guidance, to ask for His direction, and to patiently wait for the blessing He plans to bestow upon us, not in our timing, but His. But even if we make huge mistakes, we can turn back.

3. Paths we are meant to take but we don't or won't.

The Children's Bible in my dentist's office growing up had illustrations of one of the best examples of this wrong response to the right path, so much so that I can still see the picture of Jonah inside the mouth of a big fish, giant uvula hanging down in the back of its throat (although I suspect that is not anatomically correct). Perhaps the dentist used it as a prep for kids like me because after looking at that big mouth, I too was ready to say, "aaahhh" for Dr. Casino. How Jonah got there was the only part about the book that stuck with me. That is, *he ran away from the LORD* (Jonah 1:3). It only took three verses for Jonah to get to this point, so the next time you beat yourself up for not following the right path, cut yourself some slack. Perhaps that's why so many adults love this book.

What made Jonah the prophet run away in the first place was that the word of the LORD came to him with instructions to go to the great, albeit wicked, city of Nineveh and preach to the people there. (Jonah 1:1,2). Jonah's response was to run to Joppa. Not only does Jonah run away towards Joppa, but there, he boards a ship and heads precisely in the opposite direction of Nineveh towards Tarshish (modern-day Spain), planning to sail across the Mediterranean Sea to *flee from the LORD* (Jonah 1:3). Modern-day Italy would have been a considerable distance, especially for anyone who suffers from motion sickness as I do, and yet Jonah's plan is to sail as far away from Nineveh as he possibly can. Jonah does it to flee, but as a prophet, he should have known the words of the Psalmist, David, from only 200 years previously when he says, *Where can I flee from your presence? If I go up to the heavens, you are there; if I make my bed in the depths, you are there (Psalm 139: 7,8).* Still, Jonah fled, and he admitted to the sailors that he was running away from the LORD (Jonah 1:10).

Thanks to the Veggie Tales movie about and named for Jonah, and having listened to the movie as it played in my vehicle at least a *hundred times* (no exaggeration), I know that once Jonah the asparagus was tossed overboard and ended up inside the belly of a whale, there was also an amazing gospel choir inside. Through their inspirational song, *Second Chances* (sung by Anointed), the message that God is a God of second chances was conveyed to my own children better than anything I could have taught them.

So when Jonah was vomited out of the big fish and the word of the LORD came to him again, Jonah learned that obedience, the sooner the better, is the first takeaway lesson from choosing to **not** veer down this path. Jonah's obedience was somewhat pitiful and pouty. Nevertheless, the second takeaway lesson is to ask the question, "What's my Nineveh?"

Our Nineveh doesn't have to be fraught with danger to choose to resist it. Indeed, it may not look exciting or challenging enough, but the overriding message of obedience is the same.

Recently, one of our beloved youth leaders, who had a knack for getting into ridiculously challenging situations, was presented with a fork in the road that would take him to the ideal school, with an ideal scholarship, an ideal living situation, and an ideal job, but he thought that he was not meant to go that route because it almost looked too easy. He thought that unless the path was challenging and difficult, it was not the "right path." I told him I didn't know what direction he was meant to go in, but that I thought it was unfair to judge it to be the wrong path just because there were few obstacles, explaining when you run past tree stumps you see that the rings demonstrate easy years and tough years. He prayed about it and sought the Lord's direction, and has been happily fulfilled having not run away.

4. Paths we are meant to take and we take them regardless where they lead.

This is the path of obedience, and is the most difficult to learn to discern, and yet once a pattern for responding to God's leading is established, the markings on this path become more recognizable. On this path, we may be running towards something or someone or fleeing from something or someone, as Joseph did when he ran out of the house rather than be seduced by Potiphar's wife (Genesis 39).

Looking back at the forks in the road of my life, it was clear when a distinct path was before me. These were crystal clear, from the time in fifth grade when I was alone in my hospital room and felt called to choose nursing as a career path, and stayed true to that vision despite friends trying to talk me out of it. I felt the same way years later when I was running and felt called to apply for an Army ROTC scholarship for my remaining three years at Penn State.

Others were not happy with this path. My boyfriend at the time called me a "jarhead." If I had been militarily savvy I could have told him that in the Army, the term "grunt" is used, not the Marine term, "jarhead." After I had made the commitment, I once walked onto my sorority floor to a group of sisters laughing while my friend played dress up with my boots and my uniform to mock me.

Times when I have deliberately proceeded down the wrong path have been laden with red flags, and these are difficult. More difficult is when there is a path that is clear to be God's, and it's not one I have wanted to take. When my husband was in his internship year after medical school, I was working and finalizing classes to apply to medical school myself. When he found a farm for sale in 1990, I knew it was either/or. Running to a church in downtown Johnstown, I cried and cried, but knew it was God's path for us, and resolved to accept it, not knowing how clearly beneficial that decision would be to us and our children decades later.

When finally there was an opportunity to do the one thing with my nursing license I had not had the luxury to do during the twelve years my husband was in school or training, specifically to volunteer, it was glorious. I had felt called to travel to Africa for many years (probably since the harsh winter of 1977 when school was closed and we watched Alex Haley's miniseries, *Roots*). While trying to plan a mission trip, the path to Africa was thwarted, and the route to Haiti opened. When I shared with a friend that I felt God was calling me to Haiti, her response was to ask if I was sure He didn't dial the wrong number? Even the week of departure, my husband's partner said, "Have fun in Tahiti." When Jim told him that I was going to Haiti, not Tahiti, he said, "Oh no! You cannot let her go there!"

Haiti is such a unique place that once you visit, you either yearn to return to it, or yearn to flee from it. My sentiments fell into the former category. It is a complicated place that can best be understood by reading the book about Dr. Paul Farmer, *Mountains beyond Mountains*, written by Pulitzer Prize winning author Tracy Kidder.

There was a time when a medical mission trip was planned to Haiti, but the pastor who ran the church and feeding program was murdered. The team debated and assessed the potential danger. One of the doctors who had traveled many times to Haiti, Ken Van Antwerp, simply said, "If God wants me to be in Haiti, it would be a lot more dangerous place for me to be at home." The team decided and we were going. My husband and children wholeheartedly supported me in the endeavor.** Other family members were not so supportive and disapproved to the extent that they wouldn't speak to me. It wasn't that I needed their approval, but their silence was deafening. Still, it was the right path to take.

Often the response to taking the right path does not afford the luxury of indefinite time for decision. In the story of David and Goliath, David's father, Jesse, directed him to deliver food to his older brothers at the battle against the Philistines, and in immediate obedience, David *ran to the battle lines* (1 Samuel 17:22). When David bravely fought Goliath, he *ran quickly to the battle line to meet him* (1 Samuel 17:48). Perhaps that is the best lesson from the right path: when you know God wants you on it, you head immediately in that direction regardless of what others say to discourage you, even as David's older brother tried to do to him (verse 28).

You do not head to Tarshish, no matter what. The enemy will use people to thwart you from heading in the right direction.

I experienced this many times, including a time when I was planning a medical mission trip. I spent months ordering medications, booking flights for the team, planning the packing. At an exhausting time, close to our departure, there were a few church members who made me feel browbeaten, questioning whether it would be better if we just sent the trip money to the country for food and supplies, and simply cancelled the trip. Although I knew then that they were wrong, at the time I did not have the maturity to understand short-term missions to articulate the response I now know to be true. Moreover, as I tell my children, "We don't change Haiti. Haiti changes us."

If I could go back in time I could tell those who opposed our trip that short-term mission trips really aren't about the change or the good that a team can do elsewhere in the world. Short-term missions are about two things: 1) first and foremost supporting the long-term folks on the ground that work there day in and day out, and 2) changing the hearts of the members of the short term mission team to understand the communities and countries they visit and testify regarding it. And when you add the corruption with money that is prevalent in so many places you wish to help, just sending money really isn't effective without trustworthy effective people on the ground.

Years later I saw that for myself in Haiti when I witnessed the edification of Wilbert Merzilus (long term mission) by the presence of Mike Dunlap (short term mission), although the enrichment seemed mutually beneficial to Mike as well.

The last lesson about taking the right path and the most difficult to achieve is that even if it is the right path, it is important to not run ahead of God. Whether it's getting married, or moving, or taking a job or making a purchase, timing matters, and He wants us to glean insight from His teaching. 2 John 1:9 says, *"Anyone who runs ahead…does not have God…"*

My brother tells the story when he was in the Marines at Camp Lejeune, North Carolina, of a run after a week in the field eating MRE's (Meals Ready to Eat). Each brown packet contained enough calories in packets of food and dehydrated items such as fruit to survive a few days if necessary. The MRE's also could be notoriously constipating. On the first long run back from the field through trails and brush, my brother was passed as usual by the fastest member of the company. Further down the road, that same speedy soldier sped by him again. The third time this man passed him, my brother was irritated and felt like this guy was taunting him and trying to make him look bad by running ahead. He was increasingly frustrated until the revelation that this poor fellow Marine had to keep jumping into the brush to relieve himself of all those packed MRE's!

That's what I am like when I keep trying to run ahead of God. I think I can do it in my own power, and may be on the right path, sprinting ahead when I fall behind but when I fail to trust His timing, my race in life can be mightily sidetracked.

So back to having that crystal ball. Even if we had one, I think we would still find ourselves in the dark and on a wrong path from time to time. We need to remember that illumination is available.

Pondering for the Road

Which of these excerpts from Psalm 119 speak to you most?

I run in the path of your commands, for you have set my heart free. Psalm 119:32

Before I was afflicted I went astray…Psalm 119:67

I have kept my feet from every evil path so that I might obey your word. Psalm 119:101

I gain understanding from your precepts; therefore I hate every wrong path. Psalm 119:104

My Prayer for You

My prayer for you is to know that God runs too! Even when you are a long way off, having made the worst of mistakes, turn back towards Him. As soon as He sees you, he's taking off running for **you.**

Sustenance for the Road

You have made known to me the path of life; you will fill me with joy in your presence…

Psalm 16:11

How do you want to go forward?

_____

_____

_____

Do you have a story to tell about right and wrong paths? Tell it at whatilearnedwhilerunning.com.

*This camp experience occurred at an incredible Wyldlife Camp (YoungLife camp for middle schoolers), in northern Pennsylvania called Lakewood. My apologies for not knowing the names of the staff dressed up as "elderly," but if you are someone who has ever worked at any Wyldife camp, whether this one, others we have attended such as NorthBay and Michindoh, or ones we haven't attended, you are a treasure! Thank you!

** My husband was especially supportive regarding my mission trip, as he had traveled to Cambodia in 2001 to treat land-blast injuries caused by landmines that were originally planted by the Khmer Rouge during their regime ending in 1979, to keep countrymen from fleeing the country. Injuries from the mines causing loss of limb and life were still prevalent for years due to mines shifting during the rainy season. Most astonishing to my husband was the lack of the most basic provision in terms of medical care, and that the poorest in the United States were well off in comparison to most in the rest of the world.

13

Strength Training

What lies behind us and what lies before us are
tiny matters compared to what lies within us.
~Ralph Waldo Emerson

The joy of the LORD is my strength.
Nehemiah 8:10

Personal trainers will be the first to tell you that participating in just one type of exercise or activity is not ideal, including running. Even if the workout type is especially healthful, the repetition can lead to boredom and then forsaking the exercise altogether. The benefits of strength training, however, is unique in that nearly every activity and sport can be accentuated with the supplementation of this as part of the exercise regime.

Years ago, however, this was not so. In 1980, when our girls' track coach brought us into the football team's weight room, the place and purpose was an enigma at first. Indeed, weight training was thought to be for "bodybuilders." It took years for me to get on board with strength training, even after marrying a man who held the "squatting" record – yes that word/image still cracks me up – at Penn State.

What finally convicted me *should* have been the approach of my thirtieth birthday and the research at the time that suggested the benefit to women's bone density and preservation of muscle as aging occurs. Nope.

Moreover, the increase in metabolism caused by strength training as well as the toned appearance should have motivated me. Again, no.

August 1992. I traveled to Fitzsimons Army Medical Center for my two weeks of Individual Mobilization Augmentee training in the Intensive Care Unit. When I left Pennsylvania, our farm was very dry and signs at a few businesses and churches displayed, "pray for rain." Soon after I arrived in Denver, I heard there was a hurricane that would bring much needed rain to Pennsylvania, but devastation to Florida. While on post, I resided at the Officers Barracks, just down the hall from where Jim and I had stayed January through March of 1988 when we pushed the twin beds together and cooked in our room's microwave.

After in processing, my schedule involved twelve-hour shifts, so I took advantage of the time to take a 10-mile run inside post. When I returned to the barracks, another officer that was doing loops in the opposite direction from me had just finished his run, and started a conversation, because he was interested in increasing his distances, and wanted to run with me on my next long run. Obviously into strength training because of his physique, he advised me of the benefits of the same to me (because I was obviously not into strength training). He offered to orient me to the machines in the gym. Ironically, this man was a Physician's Assistant with the same name as my husband.

In the world of military camaraderie, there would have been nothing wrong with me accepting "Jim's" invitation. It sounded like fun, but I told him that I was tired and needed to take a shower and I would see how I felt afterwards, because the altitude (5,280 feet, thus "Mile-High City") always seemed to make me very exhausted after exertion. As I walked up the stairs to my room, I sensed a red flag, and I realized that familiarity of this officer in his name and medical profession was what made him seem comfortable. Certainly companionship was something that I yearned for, especially since my husband was spending up to 100 hours per week at his hospital in surgical residency. When he was home, because the nights on call involved no sleep, his home time was for sleeping and not much else. And for sure, my muscles could have used some strength training.

If you have not read the book, *The Five Love Languages*, by Gary Chapman, I implore you to do so. It will enhance your relationship or at the very least, your understanding of your relationship with virtually anyone. If you are married or are planning to be married, turn off the television, unplug electronics, and read this book aloud to one another. You will laugh heartily when you glean insights about one another, I promise! The book summarizes that each of us has one of five love languages and we express love in different ways, and appreciate love in different ways. When my husband and I read the book aloud to one another, it was one of the crucial mileposts in our marriage; we howled with laughter as we discovered each other's quirks. What we learned was that my "love language" was *Quality Time*, while his was *Physical Touch*. Now before you think every man's is physical touch, I assure you one of my friend's husband's was *Acts of Service*...so she devoted the hour prior to his arrival home from work to straightening up the house, having supper ready and fresh lipstick applied.

Unfortunately, just because you know and understand one another's love language, you cannot always meet the need to fill each other's "empty tank." When my husband was a surgical resident, it was impossible to meet my "quality time" need. But back to my story in Colorado.

When there was a knock on my door and a note pushed under, I was showered and resting on my twin bed. Because of the "red flag," I did not answer. My mantra regarding my husband was borrowed from Gladys Knight and the Pips' song, Midnight Train to Georgia, when she belts "I'd rather live with him in his world than live without him in mine." From the time I decided to marry and commit to my husband and knew that it was better to "live with him in his world than live without him in mine," the circumstances didn't change that pledge. Although this was a strictly platonic situation, and having worked in the medical profession which is a workplace ripe for being the recipient of overt romantic advances, of which I brushed off as crazily amusing, it was a defining moment in my running where I knew that no good could come of running with a man who was not my husband or a relative. This was a lesson I would carry with me for the rest of my life. On a very rare occasion in later years, I would agree in an isolated incident with a "little brother" type and when my husband was in close proximity to meet me.

This is not to criticize those who choose to run with members of the opposite sex, especially in running clubs, however there are plenty of groups of same sex runners who can be found to join in pursuit of the sport. When the illustrious career of Retired Four Star General David

Petraeus ended in scandal, with him stepping down as Director of the Central Intelligence Agency, due to scandal, my heart ached at a hero's demise. It was not a surprise that the extramarital affair with his official biographer, Paula Broadwell, developed as their mutual love of running was cited as a way time was spent together in that quest for the biography to be written. Not surprising, but disheartening nonetheless to see an American hero disgraced, and families impacted in the public arena. I am convinced the devil delights in these situations, but am strengthened to know that in addition to the knowledge that God runs toward us (Prodigal Son parable mentioned in last chapter), that the devil *flees*-**IF** we resist (James 4:7). So, the next time you face a situation, whether it is tempting or not, and you're wondering just who is in close proximity to you, remember that *God runs and the devil flees.*

Having digressed from what gave me the motivation to finally participate in strength training, rest assured it wasn't even being called out as obviously "flabby" outside those Army Officers' Quarters. No, it was a particularly personal heartbreaking occurrence not long afterwards that somehow resulted in such burning pain in my upper back, that I scheduled my first massage therapy appointment. Probably what I needed was psychotherapy when my parents split after nearly 37 years of marriage, but instead I had weekly massage therapy to cope with the pain. Adjunctively, I noticed that my legs felt fresher while running because of the massage therapy; however the relief in my back was always short-lived. When the massage therapist saw my deterioration from week to week, she recommended lifting weights to help strengthen the scapular region. As soon as I started, the pain resolved almost immediately. The takeaway lesson was twofold: how beneficial massage therapy can be to runners, especially when it is scheduled *before* painful symptoms occur and how beneficial strength training can be.

Finally! The benefits of strength training were available through my thirties, with a minimal investment of time, and it was the overall healthiest decade of my life but sadly, due to lack of adequate prioritization, my forties saw sporadic bursts. However, thanks to many popular workout videos, the masses can reap the benefits in their own homes. When our family was on a P90X kick, during a sneaky lunge sequence I remember yelling at Tony Horton on the television, (after having watched the movie

Miracle with my boys for the hundredth time-no exaggeration), "I'm Mike Eruzione, and I play for the USA!"

One of my favorite verses, *…the joy of the LORD is your strength (Nehemiah 8:10*, is certainly one to ponder). Others have noted that it does **not** say that the strength of the Lord is your joy. To scrutinize it further requires examining as to what this joy is. Is joy present happiness or delight in circumstances? Can one be joyful when happiness is elusive? According to Strong's Exhaustive Concordance, this *joy* is from the Hebrew word, *chedvah*, which means "rejoicing." So, the *rejoicing* of the LORD is your strength. Well what is the rejoicing of the LORD?

Christ the Lord has a lot to say about His joy in the 15th Chapter of the Gospel of John.

"As the Father has loved me, so have I loved you. Now remain in my love. If you obey my commands, you will remain in my love, just as I have obeyed my Father's commands and remain in his love. **I have told you this so that my joy may be in you and that your joy may be complete.** *My command is this: Love each other as I have loved you." (John 15:9-12)*

So if his joy is for us to obey his command by loving each other as we are loved, than our strength comes from this very place. Some consider it a place of weakness; they couldn't be more wrong. The Lord revealed this to Paul when he said, *"My grace is sufficient for you, for my power is made perfect in weakness."* (2 Corinthians 12:9) Loving each other is the most difficult thing in the world we are asked to do, starting within our own homes, extending outwards to our communities and nations. But if we can capitalize upon the strength of the Lord, we **will** be happy, because Psalm 84:5 says, *Blessed are those whose strength is in you.* Here is the amazing part: Blessed means *how happy!* (the exclamation point is not even mine!) How **happy** are those whose strength is in You! Still, loving requires a state of humility and servitude, so if I can grasp this, perhaps like Paul, I too can comprehend that when I am weak, then I am actually strong (2 Corinthians 12:10).

When I first knew I needed to write about strength training in this journey, and I thought about how love is extended in a community, my notes and thoughts warmly were repeatedly focused towards an organization that serves this place so many of us call home in extraordinary ways. That agency is the Community Foundation for the Alleghenies. My earliest thoughts as I started to compile my notes in 2008, were of the various funds that strengthened the community such as the Santa Fund, created for those who are in need of assistance in providing Christmas presents for their children. My own boys worked in our barn doing extra chores until they had earned one hundred dollars to give to the inaugural year of the fund. In a strange twist, it was the year my twins came home bawling because their teacher had told the class there was no such thing as Santa. (Let the record show we never said there was or wasn't a Santa. We had read books about Saint Nicholas and we always said we believe in the spirit of Santa).

After that traumatic day at school, on the front page of the paper, there was a story about a woman who had been an officer in corrections who was medically unable to work, and was unable to purchase Christmas gifts for her children without the fund. I explained to my second-graders that *they* were Santa for someone else. Other grants that improved the quality of life for people in the region included one that our local park's concession stand received in order to have running water and wheelchair accessible restrooms.

One of the things I adored most about the Foundation from the beginning was the word "for" rather than "of," because it describes perfectly that it embodies those on the giving side as well as receiving, and most people have the opportunity to readily embrace both sides. It all happened because of the vision of Richard Mayer, a distinguished citizen who made innumerable contributions to the Johnstown region. He is not known nationally, but should be for founding the Community Foundation and serving as chairman for 12 years. He was an excellent role model for the current board chair, Mark Pasquerilla, the son of a successful and wealthy businessman who perpetuates his parents' philanthropic spirit and inspires the community to continue to invest in a region that others at one time thought was forsaken.

Since my earliest notes (and I haven't shared with anyone that I have written about the Foundation), I was coincidentally asked to be on the Marketing Committee. Since I have no marketing background or expertise, and since the staff humbly, efficiently, and creatively convey the Foundation's message, I suspect it is my very talkative nature in conveying to others my enthusiasm for things I embrace that put me in that role, although some might find my fervor annoying without a doubt. Indeed, as years have gone by, I could weep at all the ways life is enhanced for nearly everyone in an extended area- from all socioeconomic backgrounds- whether through scholarships, clean water initiatives, recreation projects, 4th of July concerts...the list is endless. I would be remiss **not** to testify that involvement for *anyone* conveys to me how joy gives strength.*

Pursuing strength is a worthwhile pursuit. However there is one type of lifting that we are **not** meant to bear and that is false guilt. For the longest time, I felt guilty that the first thing I sat down and read every morning was Oswald Chamber's *My Utmost For His Highest*. This went on for years. The burden I bore was guilt that I didn't read scripture first. Finally, when it was time to confess, the person whom I knew would speak truth and love to me was Muff Dunlap, and I released my burden over tea and soup, awaiting her wisdom, advice, and admonishment. She set down her spoon, raised her eyebrows and exclaimed, "That's what Mike does! He says, 'It primes the pump!'" The burden I had been bearing was a false burden, meant to drag me down. We are not meant to lift these types of weights. So if you are dealing with guilt, I beg you to find someone of counsel you can trust, willing to accept direction, but also willing to accept that perhaps the enemy has been enlisting you to bear a burden that you *aren't* meant to carry, a burden of *false guilt*, then let it go.

As for me, on this journey, as my recovery from back surgery (from the herniated disc mentioned in the introduction) allows more latitude from activity restrictions, (I am now permitted to lift ten pounds), I *need* yet another treasure from the twelfth chapter of Hebrews, the reminder of this: *Therefore, strengthen your feeble arms and weak knees* (Hebrews 12:12). How about you? Do you also need to pursue getting stronger one way or another, or are you in a place where you are hurting so badly, you just need a massage? Even in weakness, I have learned I can be strong and courageous, even if just to muster enough strength to take care of myself, and schedule a workout or even that massage in order to continue to draw strength that enables me to go on the heights.

Pondering for the Road

What strength training do you need? Are you drawing from the source of strength mentioned in Habakkuk 3:19? *The Sovereign Lord is my strength; he makes my feet like the feet of a deer, he enables me to go on the heights.*

My Prayer for You

My prayer for you is that if you need to be strengthened, that you would ***know*** *that the words from Philippians 4:13 apply to you this day:* I can do all things through Christ who strengthens me.

Sustenance for the Road

The name of the LORD is a strong tower; the righteous run to it and are safe. Proverbs 18:10

(Proverbs 18:10)

How do you want to go forward?

_____

_____

_____

Tell your strength training experience at whatilearnedwhilerunning.com.

*Disclaimer: With humility and honor, I began a term on the board of the Foundation in 2015 just as this book is going to print; whole books should be written about the positive continual influence of this organization upon the Pennsylvania counties of Cambria, Somerset, and Bedford, and the small investment is now well over 50 million dollars.

Colleen Tretter

140

14

Love and Prejudice

Darkness cannot drive out darkness: only light can do
that. Hate cannot drive out hate: only love can do that.
~Martin Luther King, Jr.

Love the Lord your God with all your heart and with all your
soul and with all your mind. Love your neighbor as yourself.
Matthew 22:37,39

God has taught me many things on this journey, but it took a long time
to learn that I am prejudiced. It took many miles of toil and many prayers
for revelation, but the fact remains that He clearly revealed to me that I am
prejudiced. The seeds of it were inadvertently planted in childhood, and
somehow it grew and flourished. Now you may be thinking the prejudice
of which I speak is racial prejudice but no, that's not it.

At the time of my first draft, it seemed racial prejudice still is a volatile
issue in this nation. Perhaps by the time this manuscript is complete, it
won't be so. Many white people don't realize how profound prejudice is.
Having lived in Hawaii was a blessing for the obvious reason that it is an
amazingly beautiful paradise. However, the lessons and insights gleaned
there were invaluable, such as taking off your shoes without exception
upon entering a home, and not honking your horn, unless absolutely
necessary. Once, while I was jogging in place at an intersection, I watched
as a driver of a vehicle, waiting behind another vehicle whose driver missed

the green light, waited until that driver looked up and *never* honked his horn. Hawaiian time could wait. Negative experiences while living there also taught inestimable understanding.

When I worked in a non-military hospital in 1988, it was clear that Caucasian nurses were not held in as high regard as those of Polynesian and Asian descent. There was even a racial slur for white people- the "h" word, although when we returned in 1997, it was politically incorrect enough to suggest that there was an effort to eradicate it. However, when I was in the regular community, I would notice for example, that even if I was next in line at a deli counter, a man of Asian descent would be waited on first. My status was elevated when my son, Paul, was with me among local women because of his dark skin. "Aww, you married local boy, ya?" None of this even compares to the racial injustices African American and American Indian people have endured for centuries in our country, but I honestly believe if people could experience prejudice even in a mild form, it would be a great learning experience.

Conversely, transcending to a state of being *loved* despite the color of your skin is by far one of life's greatest moments of bliss, something that I also experienced in Hawaii from a circle of quilters at the Queen Emma Summer Palace, taught by John and Poakalani Serrao.* I had always wanted to learn how to quilt in the traditional American way, but never had the opportunity to learn. When I learned the Hawaiian way, I fell in love with the tradition, and was embraced by the Serrao family to the extent that John made me an original design of two dolphins when I was pregnant with my twin boys. Even though I lacked skill compared to other quilters, mistakes were reminders from my teachers that "only God is perfect." If a quilter had a flawless piece, which was never my problem, a 'flaw' would be added. Oh to sit in that circle and listen to them 'talk story' and discuss the annual hula competition, the Merry Monarch Festival! Those ladies (and John) probably don't even remember my white face, but through that Hawaiian quilting, I felt *loved*.

The journey to learning about my prejudice was slow and arduous. When the epiphany about the *joy of the LORD* (previous chapter) so captivated me, the pursuit of the command to *Love one another* resounded in my head. Nearly every religion in a pure uncorrupted form embraces this mandate, and yet as a global society we fail so miserably. The "love" passage from 1 Corinthians 13 is a traditional reading at weddings, but only 6 percent of marriages last 50 years according to the last census. If we have difficulty with our spouse, the one person with whom we choose to spend the rest of our life, no wonder we struggle with love when it comes to our siblings, mothers, neighbors, and dare I say it, in-laws, let alone strangers. So my quest was to discover specifically why I fail in the command to *love one another.* My New Year's resolution/prayer in 2006 was for God to help me love as He loves, and like many who fail, found myself right back to where I was December 31ˢᵗ, but could not figure out why until I discovered my severe prejudice.

The beginning of my comprehending came that following December at a military funeral for a Marine who died in Afghanistan. He was the husband of one of the "mommy" friends in the group of women, babies and toddlers who gathered together in Hawaii. I wanted my three older sons to accompany me to the burial in Arlington to grasp the magnitude of sacrifice for our freedom, but it was I who grasped something else.

As we left the church of Trane McCloud's funeral, across the street were protesters holding signs that read, "GOD HATES HOMOSEXUALS." I had only just learned about this group who attributed the deaths of our service personnel to our nation's evolving accepting stance on homosexuality. So they would show up at military funerals and protest loudly in front of grieving families. My sons saw them and asked what they were shouting, and my oldest son read their signs. When they asked me to explain, all I could say was, "That is what hatred looks like, not what being a Christian should look like."

Let the record show that I am not sharing any opinion regarding homosexuality, but I admit that the in the AIDS crisis, homosexual patients were those I had no problem caring for as a registered nurse. Truthfully, when I traveled from New York to Hawaii, I welcomed caring for AIDS patients as a result of homosexual transmission, because the patients and visitors who were IV drug abusers in New York were brutal in terms of making staff worry about sharps containers, narcotics, manipulation etc. One of my favorite patients in Hawaii, "Randy," (of Portuguese descent) whom I cared for as my own brother while his partner languished in grief nearby, blessed me in getting to know his family, including his brother, who introduced non-native nurses such as myself to "malasadas" or Portuguese doughnuts that became my motivation for hiking Diamond Head frequently (Leonard's Bakery was just down the hill).

Back to the sign holders outside the funeral of the serviceman who died defending their right to free speech...when it comes to the Great Commission, if where God wants us is the North Pole, these types of people are on the South Pole. They in fact repel the message of love from being heard in polar opposition. Unfortunately, when I find myself hating these people with a purple passion, suddenly I transport myself to the ***exact*** same location. I think I'll see polar bears, but wonder, "How did these penguins get here?"

Schadenfreude is a German word that shockingly has no English equivalent. It means to delight in bad things happening to others. The whole tabloid industry virtually depends upon those deriving pleasure from others' pain. However, when I am astonished by that person with a Christian fish magnet who cuts me off in traffic, then I become indignant as the vehicle speeds by, then am delighted when I see the police lights emerge on to the highway ahead of me to pull the vehicle over, I have pitifully become a "Schadenfreuder (my word)."

2013...Another year and the same resolution. *Crazy Love*, a remarkable book and study by Francis Chan, was insightful and moving, yet my heart was still saying, "Help me love as You love." Beth Moore's Deuteronomy study on the "Law of Love," was also enlightening; nonetheless, I had fallen short again. Maybe I should just be like other people and resolve to lose weight January first. Finally, as another year heralded an enlightening run south on Route 601, that broken place was reached and I found myself asking, "Why am I failing miserably in trying to love like You love? And that's when He laid it on my heart...*the Good Samaritan*. What *about* the Good Samaritan? As a child, it was one of the parables I always enjoyed hearing in church on Sundays as the gospel reading, because there were some, quite frankly that scared me to high heaven like the Parable of the Loaned Money (Matthew 25). (It seemed completely logical to me to hide the talent in the ground. I remember thinking, "Yikes!" when the master called the man a wicked lazy servant, and he was tossed outside into the darkness).

Almost everyone knows the story about the Good Samaritan, even though this teaching parable only appears in the tenth chapter of the gospel of Luke. Agencies are named after this fictitious person, even hospitals (I worked in one). On that chilly day, I rushed home to scour every word. To summarize, an expert in the law tests Jesus about what he must do to inherit eternal life, but by doing so answers himself as he recites Deuteronomy 6:5 and Leviticus 9:18, that he reads the law to mean, "Love the Lord your God with all your heart and with all your soul and with all your strength and with all your mind, and 'Love your neighbor as yourself.'"(Luke 10:27). But then this expert asks Jesus the question, "And who is my neighbor?" (Luke 10:29).

So Jesus tells the parable with the gist of the story being that there is a man who is beaten, robbed, and left half dead in the road. A priest and a Levite, the expert in the religious law, pass him by. The Samaritan (the scourge of society to the Israelites) is the one who helps him and brings him to an inn where he pays the manager to take care of him and promises to come back and pay anything extra. Jesus tells this parable to the expert in the law to define just who is our neighbor.

At the end of the parable, Jesus asks that expert which of the three men in the story was a neighbor to the man, and the expert answers, *The one who had mercy on him"(Luke 10:37)*

On New Year's Day, I realized this parable is really a story about more than three people, but specifically which type of person I have difficulty loving.

First, there is obviously the man. Then there are the robbers. Next, there is the priest and the Levite, the Samaritan, and the innkeeper. Quite possibly there was a doctor after the fact, as well as someone to bring this man clothing and food, but we aren't told that. I remember a sermon that painted an image of this man whom the Samaritan found "in the gutter" and my childhood brain mistakenly translated that he was possibly homeless or somehow lived in that condition. Regardless, I could love him. I don't know why but I could even love the robbers. Obviously I could love the Samaritan. Even though the innkeeper took payment to help this man, I could also love him. But here is the key to my problem regarding loving: I do not love the priest and the Levite. This is my prejudice, and my hurdle to overcome.

In my defense, having *stood* through each Passion Sunday liturgy year after year after year, and hearing that Jesus told his disciples that he was going to suffer thanks to the hands of the elders, chief priests, and teachers of the law, and *be killed* (Matthew 16:21), and *especially* that they plotted killing him after Lazarus was raised from the dead, well these were hateful people that I believe I started hating as a child.

The illumination was finally shown on the realization that nearly all of my negative unloving emotions towards others I had difficulty loving were those I perceived to be self-righteous "Pharisees." I remember thinking after a particularly brutal comment by a Christian woman after a sermon including the verse from John 14:2, *In my Father's house there are many rooms...*, "Lord, please let me be on a different wing, or at the very least don't let us share an elevator!" However, I knew in my heart that with God's sense of humor, these very people most likely would be my roommate, or at the very least, share a balcony!

The veil was finally lifted for me. Christ died for **everyone** in that parable. Not just for the man beaten, or the Samaritan, or the innkeeper, but for **everyone.** Even the priest. Even the Levite...THAT is the love that has been elusive to me. He died for every one...every last one of us. He loves even the self-righteous who could ignore someone in need. Because I never want to forget where grace found me, when others act hateful and above grace, my heart has reacted unlovingly. *All* have merit in His eyes. My prejudice had to go. It has to go. That is my daily struggle to love as He loves. So the question I have for you is this, "Who in the parable of the Good Samaritan do you have difficulty loving as God loves?" Someone you might perceive as greedy? Someone you perceive as in the gutter or beneath you? Someone you have a prejudice against? A "Samaritan," perhaps?

If this isn't earth shattering to you, you must have no difficulty loving indeed. A test regarding love of self is easy: you need look no further than what Tom Clancy identified as an "I love me wall," in one of his novels, where one displays every certificate and accolade for all to see like a shrine (unless you are looking at a physician, lawyer, or other office wall where those types of items need to be displayed).

A good test regarding love for others would be to imagine if you could fulfill Jesus' teaching from Matthew 5:41. *"If someone forces you to go one mile, go with him two miles."* (I'm not talking about actual distances, you know, so don't lace up just yet). One of the most striking images to convey this verse is in the photographic masterpiece, *Journeys with the Messiah,* by

Michael Belk, a fashion photographer who felt called to use his talent and creativity to demonstrate the present-day relevance of Christ. In the *Second Mile* photograph, you will literally gasp as you see Jesus walking alongside a Nazi. A Nazi! Nazis are the one group we are allowed to hate, right? An entire video game capitalized on this called "Nazi Zombies." Nazis did heinous things that should not be forgotten. But Christ turns our views upside down, and Belk captures that beautifully. All of the images are captivating, but this one poignantly so.

So once the resolve to love is there, could the next step be taken? Could I spur on a Pharisee? We are to *spur one another on*, according to Hebrews 10.

Let us hold unswervingly to the hope we profess, for he who promised is faithful. And let us consider how we may spur one another on toward love and good deeds (Hebrews 10:23,24). If I can spur another on, would that person perhaps stop to help the man beaten and robbed? What if it's a child who has not been loved-could his path of say, becoming a robber be redirected? Could overcoming the prejudice and loving as I should create a better world? Yes! Of course! The key is unlocked, but still not simple. Knowing isn't doing. But I have learned my weakness, especially when my children are in the crossfire of the self-righteous. When a Christian man tells my fourteen year-old son that, "Those people who run with shorts, well there's no way they are going to heaven," my head confirms the 212 phenomenon regarding steam, because I'm sure I look like 'Yosemite Sam,' fumes pouring out my ears (not because I run in shorts, but because this Phariseeism was shared with a minor).

I still remember when believers told my young children that they "worshipped Satan" because they went trick or treating in my mother's neighborhood. I was indignant because they weren't dressed like a horror Freddie Kruegger; they were giraffes or cows! Still, when I react this way, I then find myself in the same position as the Rich Young Ruler who *ran* up to Jesus (Mark 10:17) seeking truth, receiving it with the all important directive from Christ in Matthew's version of this encounter to "Love your neighbor as yourself," (Matthew 19:19), and still going away empty. Even after having been genuinely *loved* as he was loved (Mark 10:21). My foot slips at times like these.

Again and again we are called to die to self, but when we fail, we can remember this... *When I said, "My foot is slipping," your love, O LORD, supported me. (Psalm 94:18).*

147

The fact of the matter is that we will slip as long as we have emotions. We don't have to be teenagers to have joy, pain and drama. We only have to be alive. One of my favorite passages about the emotions of Christ comes from *The Relationship Principles of Jesus* by Tom Holladay.

> *Consider the way Jesus is often pictured in movies-wandering through the countryside in a kind of daze, as though he has no feelings whatsoever about what's going on around him.*
>
> *This false picture causes us to equate spiritual strength with being emotionally distant. The message many of us hear is, "The more you deny your emotions, the more you will be like Jesus."*
>
> *Yet when you look at Jesus' life, you see a man filled with emotion. You see his emotion in his tender compassion for a man ravaged by leprosy (Mark 1:40-42). You experience the depth of his feelings in his wrenching distress as he prays in Gethsemane about his impending death on the cross (Mark 14:33). You feel the emotion of gentle love Jesus has for his mother as he speaks to her from the cross (John 19:26-27).*

The apostle Peter learned this lesson about emotions well, and when he was able to get over his prejudice towards Gentiles, he created a layered parfait of his own topped with love in his epistle. (2 Peter 1:5-7- I'll let you look that one up.)

So this is it. Chairō, a Greek word that is a salutation upon greeting or departing (reminds me so much of "aloha"), meaning "God speed," is the inspiration for what I need.

What I need is a starting gun for my own First Corinthians 13.

1 Corinthians 13 for The Race

If I cheer for those running the race, but have not love, I'm just another loud spectator.

If I convey all understanding that others have taught me and I have learned about the sport of running, and glean understanding to the mysteries of the perseverance of faith, but don't have love, I am just another coach.

If I clean all the garbage along the sides of the road, but don't have love, I am just another trash hauler.

If I surrender my body to training and justify that it is a temple, but neglect my loved ones indefinitely in doing so, I have gained nothing but a shell.

If I give water to those who thirst, but have not love, I'm just another volunteer.

If I run full-sprint to rescue someone for a righteous cause, I may be a first responder. But with love, I am a servant with a higher power.

If I only love some in the race, and not all, I'm just a partial fan.

I may fail in my race, but love doesn't. Love… is the finish line.

So here I am with all I have to offer. Before, it was life living *for fear that I was running or had run my race in vain. (Galatians 2:2)* It would have been the case if the veil had not been lifted. When I run, I want to be like Mary Magdalene on Easter morning, when she discovered the empty tomb and *came running* to Simon Peter and John, trying to find the Lord. (John 20:2). Because of her, Peter and John started *running,* too (and of course, since they're men, it had to involve a footrace where one outran the other. Yes, John, we know you came in first and beat Peter to the tomb)!

All this manuscript may be is a simple act of obedience in having completed it, so that I can say, "I have fought the good fight!" And that would be enough for me. I can sleep at night with no nagging guilt of disobedience. I can begin Downton Abbey Season 3, and finally clean my closet! Or not. I can definitely begin Downton Abbey.

But if by sharing this manuscript, I arouse others to take off on their own journey, even if it is only a physical one, then perhaps that is enough. If, however, while they are sojourning, He is sought, then I can say, "I have finished the race, I have kept the faith." (2 Timothy 4:7)

Chairō. God speed.

Pondering for the Road

Do you have a prejudice? Are you willing to fight through it? When was the last time you could say that you have fought the good fight? Scripture doesn't say, "Blessed are the peacekeepers." Christ says, "Blessed are the peacemakers."(Matthew 5:9)

My Prayer for You

*My prayer for you is to not languish as long as I did trying to identify the people you have difficulty loving. And if you are the type who has difficulty loving **anyone**, take heart! **You** are not the person **I** have difficulty loving!*

Sustenance for the Road *(this version of this verse is from a beautiful book given to my children entitled* Who Made God? *By Larry Libby)...*

May you have power with all God's people to understand Christ's love. May you know how wide and long and high and deep it is. And may you know his love, even though it can't be known completely. Then you will be filled with everything God has for you. Ephesians 3:18-19

How do you want to go forward?

_____

_____

_____

Share your experience regarding love at whatilearnedwhilerunning.com

*Poakalani has an amazing story, part of which revolves around how she started teaching Hawaiian quilting. She told me that when John was away in the military, she was struggling financially to provide for her daughters. As I remember her story, at night she kept dreaming that the answer was in her closet. Her closet was where quilts were stored, including her grandmother's. Since it's taboo for a "true" quilter to sell the quilts (with

Hawaiian aloha, you give them as gifts), she was mystified. Then it came to her that she could teach others to quilt, and through that the business was formed.

Ti leaf quilt: My first piece and one that John convinced me to frame despite the uneven spacing in quilting, because I was pregnant with my twins and my finger-width changed throughout the day because of swelling. Ti leafs have been used in cooking, for spiritual blessings, for medicinal purposes, and when wrapped around a rock, can be left on a trail to alert others that someone is on the trail (and also to help as a marker to prevent getting lost).

15

The First Chapter

I was sixteen in October 1981, during what should have been my senior year of high school, but school was not in session. We had not attended school since the week after Memorial Day. There was a teachers' strike, or more descriptively, a battle royale between the school board and teachers' union. Everything seemed surreal, including how I had gotten to this place.

My mother's knitting needles clicked nearby as she worked. If I could have rocked back and forth in my chair, I would have, but I was frozen. My mind was trying to process the despair I was feeling.

I wished I could go back in time to the day the year started for me. Not on New Year's Day, but during Christmas break of my junior year, on my sixteenth birthday. A group of high schoolers, including my older brother and his friends as well as my boyfriend, went sled riding at a park not far from our home. It was cold. Ronald Reagan was President, and had survived after having been shot earlier in the year. When the pope was shot just months after Reagan, some of the kids in my school said the apocalypse was coming.

My own world seemed to slowly unfurl ever since a dark December morning in 1976 when I went down to the kitchen as a seventh grader expecting my mom to be there as I had breakfast and found the completely unexpected. My dad. He slowly and gently tried to tell me that something had happened to the love of my life at that time. Something had happened to the one person who made me feel I was special. My grandmother had died.

She wasn't a perfect woman, I knew, but oh how I loved when she hugged me. Her own mother had died in the flu epidemic of 1919, leaving her to be in charge of a household with a Serbian father who could not speak English, and her brothers.

My grandmother was hard on my mother. I remember her saying, "Elaine, this oven is filthy." My mother was an only child trying to raise six kids. She took in her cousins for a summer when their parents divorced. She rarely talked about the time when I was in the hospital as a baby with pneumonia in 1965, except to talk about the nurse, Rosemary Belak who held me when my mother was not even permitted in the unit. She hadn't expected me to live, and I think the fear that I would die never left her, perhaps to the point that she could not get too emotionally attached to me. Life was tough for her. My father traveled a lot. On one occasion I remember my grandma helping my mom clean the bedrooms. My mother was crying. I didn't understand her exhaustion and weariness but I heard her say to her mother, "Mom, I'm just so tired." When I asked why my mom was crying, they wouldn't elaborate.

When my grandmother died, her father, my great-grandfather was grief-stricken. We called him, "Tut" and the only word he ever said to me that I understood was "babushka," as he patted my cheek and handed me a silver dollar. He wailed at the funeral home words I didn't understand, and everyone cried. My mom said the most unnatural thing for any parent is for their child to die first.

Our home was even more chaotic after my grandma died because my mom had the extra responsibility of looking after her disabled father, and moving her grandfather to her uncle's home.

Still, my friends envied my household, with parents who were active in the church, and chaos that comes with six kids who were athletic, smart, and involved in many activities. Our home was open to others, even if they raided our freezer of Christmas cookies and peanut-butter balls (we were Pennsylvanians, so we didn't make "buckeyes").

It wasn't anyone's fault that I didn't feel really loved by someone but my own, but that's how I felt. I was happy delivering newspapers and running errands for the neighbors to the bakery, deli, and five and dime store. I had food to eat, clothes to wear, and books to read. Every family on the street had at least five children, so we all had a blast sled-riding in winter and being outside in summer until "the streetlights turned on. Some parents of large families believed "God will provide;" others believed that "God is too busy to worry about this family."

Six months after my grandmother's death, on July 5, 1977, my brother and one of the kids who was at our house so much he could confuse a census taker, came to the local playground where I was biding time waiting for my out of state cousins to arrive. They came to order me home. When I became hysterical with fear that something had happened to one of our dogs, my brother revealed the truth. Our uncle and aunt had died in a car accident in Hazleton. Our four cousins who were in the Volkswagen van were alive, but two were badly hurt.

The word of the summer repeated over and over again was tragedy. People talked about how long the funeral procession was. There were enough flower arrangements to cover floats in a parade. Yet, when my cousins came to live with us, and share the bedroom my younger sister and I shared, it didn't feel tragic. We played backgammon under the pine trees and spades on the back porch while the radio played the Bee Gees. My mom bought us Tickle anti-perspirant in blue, pink and yellow so we could tell which one was ours. I remember one night when my mom came into my room as I was sleeping on the floor and said she was proud of me for how I was handling everything, and that she loved me.

But then my cousins went to live with another aunt and uncle who had no children, so that they and their brothers would not be divided between two families who already had six children. And I was alone. Again.

So a few years later, when my boyfriend and I started dating, it felt like the true love and companionship I had been waiting for all my life, had arrived. I don't know why we were fighting on my 16th birthday. We had a great Christmas together. I had been irritable with him ever since he was bragging about his new pool table. As I had taken a shot in a corner pocket, I heard him say that it was expensive but that his dad chewed them down.

"What do you mean he "chewed" them down?"

"Not chewed. Jew'ed. You know," he replied, "how Jewish people are."

I held the pool stick and just stared at him, and then too loudly said, "What are you talking about?" He tried to explain; I continued to be uncomprehending, having never before heard that prejudice. Immediately I thought of the one childhood friend who had the opportunity to bring me to her synagogue, and although it was unfamiliar, I thoroughly enjoyed going with her and her family. So the more furious I got, the more frustrated my boyfriend was with me for not agreeing or understanding. We left for sled riding in a huff.

How we got onto the subject of sex, I'm not sure, but my boyfriend was pointing out the couples that were "doing it." The night deteriorated into an argument when I emphatically said our relationship was not going "there." He told me he loved me and couldn't continue indefinitely that way and he broke up with me on my sixteenth birthday. He dropped me off at my house and I cried myself to sleep.

Looking back as an adult and all I know now about recognizing inherent values in people, I should have said, "good riddance." But I was beyond devastated, and had no one to whom I could confide, except a male high school friend who knew what had happened. He told me my boyfriend would come back and apologize, which he did. If you are a teenage girl and reading this, the lesson here is *don't take him back.* Which is what I did.

Months went by and I held my ground, but then I eventually gave in to him. When fall began, my parents traveled every weekend to my brother's college football games. There was no school, no Homecoming to anticipate because of the teacher's strike. I started running to the cemetery where my aunt and uncle were buried near my other grandmother.

I don't know what exactly made my mom suspicious to the extent that she tore my closet apart and found the pregnancy test I had purchased, but hadn't used. She confronted me and was immensely angry and disappointed. I was grounded in my room. When I heard her talking on the phone downstairs, I unscrewed the receiver and removed the piece that picked up the sound, held my finger over the dial tone button and gently lifted it to hear her conversation. She was speaking with our family physician, a kind, gentle and compassionate Korean immigrant, whom she trusted completely.

I heard him telling her in his sing song broken English, "Young gorls have vewy difficult time..uh. because pelvis not wide enough.....Dey can die giving birth. I was numb and waited until they finished the conversation to hang up the phone and put it back together. Then I crept back to my room.

My mom came to tell me that they were taking me to see a doctor, and I asked if it was our doctor. She said no. We ended up at Planned Parenthood. At first I was relieved, until they escorted me beyond the locked door of the waiting room to a room to undress and give a urine sample, then to an exam room and while I awaited my first pelvic exam, talked to me about abortion. I told them I didn't believe in it and neither did my boyfriend. I started to panic, as they were telling me all kinds of statistics, and why my life would be ruined if I didn't go to college (I had already been accepted and already had enough credits to graduate even though I was sixteen). They showed me pamphlets about how in earliest stages there isn't even a heartbeat. My head was swirling, and I felt completely caged. And then a reprieve: the doctor came in to say that the pregnancy test was negative. I prayed that it would be so, and they told my mom to bring me back the following week.

My parents allowed me to speak to my boyfriend on the phone, and I told him everything that had happened, and that they were taking me back there the following week. He was panicked too, and we brainstormed whom we could turn to for help, but there was no one. He promised to figure something out and that he would come for me before the following appointment. I have never prayed so hard in my life.

The night before the appointment, I listened for a sound at my window. I was ready with a bag to jump out to him. He never came. We went to the appointment, and I half expected him to meet us there, but he didn't. This is where I sat wanting to rock back and forth to the beat of my mom's knitting needles. I was taken beyond the locked door down the hallway with the same procedure as the week before. Only this time the test came back positive. I told them my boyfriend said he was going to meet me. They repeated the information they had given me the previous week and told me that my parents wanted what was best for me and my life and that we shouldn't wait because the "earlier the better." I asked if my mom could come back, and they told me no, only patients could be there. I cried and wanted to be rescued. But I was half naked and alone. Forsaken. The next hour was a blur. I wanted to die.

The next months I was dead inside. The first full week of school was in November. I was in crowds, but isolated. In school, but utterly empty. I continued to run to the cemetery. Sometimes I sat next to the grave on the cold ground. The only thing that made me feel alive was running, which was why I decided to finally run in the Trot for Tots. There was no one to rescue me. Through running, my journey with God began. He rescued me.

Years later as I was walking with my mom I finally asked her why she and my dad had brought me to that place. She told me that if I had run out and refused, she would have accepted that and dealt with it. I thought back to having been naked from the waist down behind a locked door with my clothes across the hall. And I realized that she was right. I was only sixteen, but it was all my own fault. No one else's. I didn't run. From that day forward, I knew I was never going to not run *toward someone who was in need or alone. I was never going to* not run *and take a stand in something I believed, even if it meant I would be humiliated.*

I wasn't going to include this chapter in this manuscript, but had it ready to tell the truth for those who would malign me for writing about faith. God laid it on my heart to include it. I know He forgives my past and is with me in my present. I trust Him to secure my future. Still, it wasn't easy. I hadn't shared this with hardly anyone since I shared with my husband when we first started dating. He revealed his true character of love like a vast ocean where you cannot fathom its depth. I had recently felt led to share it with the Dunlaps, and Mike asked why I hadn't shared it before. He asked if I was concerned people would think less of me, and I told him no, that no one could think less of me than I have thought about myself in my life.

I realized I wanted to protect my parents from the heartache of remembering that difficult time, and from any responsibility. It was my responsibility. I accept that. Why God wanted me to include this, I don't know. Perhaps there is someone who feels completely alone and forsaken, and I would love to share that it's not true! You are not deserted. You are loved.

I had prayed for clarity regarding including this chapter one morning. Two days prior, in the car on the way to school with three of my boys, we had a conversation about peacocks. I don't know why we started talking about them, (maybe because we had them outside our apartment in Hawaii). I told the boys I would really like to have peacocks someday. I asked them if they thought peacocks would stick around if we got some when they were very young. My youngest son told me that there are white peacocks that people really want, and they pulled up a picture for me, because I thought he meant an albino peacock.

So later that day that I had prayed for clarity, (two days after that conversation) two things happened. The first was that two peacocks showed up at our farm: a beautiful blue male with all the traditional magnificence, and a precious delicate white female. The second was that I was at my son's high school state playoff game and a bystander was hit in the face with a foul ball, and he went down. Before I could think, I ran from the bleachers to him.

It still wasn't easy to include this chapter. But those peacocks have stayed, and the female is sitting on four eggs as I type these last few sentences. God is alive. I say again, "Chairō. God speed."

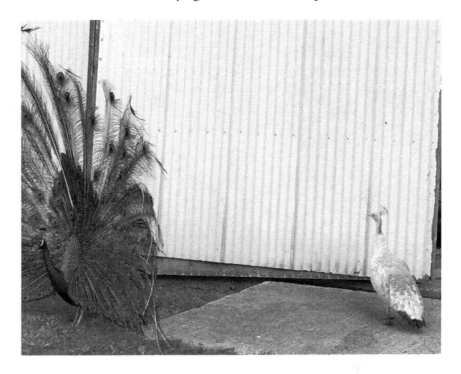

ACKNOWLEDGEMENTS

Three individuals have influenced me most on my spiritual journey, and perhaps I will only be able to properly thank them on the other side of heaven, especially because one of them is already there. Dr. Charles Stanley, Beth Moore and Oswald Chambers have blessed me for many years, from my baby steps to my stumbles and falls. Any sure strides I have run in the right direction towards the Father, Son and Holy Spirit can be attributed to these spiritual giants humbly and lovingly pointing the way. Any insights from this expedition that resonate properly are to their credit; those with dissonance are mine alone.

In terms of running, Sheron Watson, my gym teacher in high school (renowned for her volleyball coaching prowess), was the first to challenge me beyond mere sprints to longer distances in first period runs through dewy grass fields, sparking a flame that was kindled by my trigonometry teacher, Tom Shirley. My track coaches, Jay and Geary Tray, were kind and honorable, but did not realize that when I relinquished my senior year season, running was my means of survival, so I slipped through their fingers like sand.

This book would not have been completed without the encouragement and editing of my son, Cooper, who diligently helped with his "Nooooo!" comments and "what?" highlights. Then, when the crisis came, and I tried to delete the whole project, it was Paul, my sweet boy who hugged me and made me promise to finish it. He also knew how to make me laugh when he said he didn't want to read it just now but he wanted the first and only bound book.

My dear friends, Muff Dunlap and Cindy West, were kind enough to preview a few chapters, but more importantly are always there when I need, coming alongside me when my race is isolated. Mike Dunlap assisted me tremendously with Chapter 11. Autumn Battaglia, one of my favorite nurses, gave valuable feedback to the entire project, and me a great chuckle at Mike's question regarding the word eliminating, "Is that code for going to the bathroom?" Yes, Mike it is indeed.

Mike Kane, President and Executive Director of The Community Foundation for the Alleghenies, was essential in correcting my course with regard to the history of this great organization, and his accessibility is appreciated more than he can know.

Our godchild and my favorite "editor" since her college days at Penn State, Jessica White Harbin, took time from her own work and busy life as a wife of a Navy officer, and mother of two young children (need I say more), to demonstrate she still has an eye for detail, readying the entire manuscript, and giving me feedback that was invaluable.

The ladies who came to my home Wednesday mornings for six years, especially Kathy Carney, Annie Dachille, Parveen Nathaniel, Ellen Daniels, amongst those who came and went, blessed me beyond measure as we shared coffee and tears, studied God's Word, and learned to become "Mordecais" for one another. Then, when I was led to stop hosting- not knowing why-they supported me in my obedience, and thus this project was finally completed. Not having them week after week felt like the lonely stretch of the Marine Corps Marathon, but it was a portion of my journey I had to go through alone. Now that they are present at the Thursday afternoon study at the Outreach building, it feels as though I am back amongst the great cloud of witnesses.

Lexi Miller (now Marks), our blessed babysitter who was my fine line between sanity and insanity, allowed me the freedom to run all those years someone was in diapers!

Lastly, without my husband Jim, who became the most dedicated physician I have ever met, despite the fact that I tried to talk him out of achieving his dream, I could never have completed the 30,000 miles, or survived the hills and valleys with as much joy as I have had. While it was a long road, (4 years of medical school, 1 year of internship, 5 years of surgical residency, 2 years of vascular surgery fellowship, and 4 years of Army active duty), his work ethic and stamina is unequaled, and I could not proceed with any of my pursuits without his encouragement of my dreams.

Made in the USA
Middletown, DE
04 October 2015